General Practice Today

Today
A Practical Guide to Modern Consultations

General Practice Today
A Practical Guide to Modern Consultations

Dr Jane Wilcock

BSc, FRCGP, PGCertMedEd, MAHEd, SFHEA
GP Silverdale Medical Practice, Salford CCG
Year assessment lead and community clinical tutor
University of Liverpool School of Medicine

Illustrations by
Grace Mutton

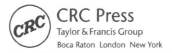

CRC Press
Taylor & Francis Group
Boca Raton London New York

CRC Press is an imprint of the
Taylor & Francis Group, an **informa** business

CRC Press
Taylor & Francis Group
6000 Broken Sound Parkway NW, Suite 300
Boca Raton, FL 33487-2742

© 2018 by Taylor & Francis Group, LLC
CRC Press is an imprint of Taylor & Francis Group, an Informa business

No claim to original U.S. Government works

Printed in Great Britain by Ashford Colour Press Ltd

International Standard Book Number-13: 978-1-1380-3573-7 (Paperback)

Visit the Taylor & Francis Web site at
http://www.taylorandfrancis.com

and the CRC Press Web site at
http://www.crcpress.com

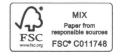

Contents

Introduction

There are lots of different ways of consulting in general practice, and there are a myriad of factors which weigh in those consultations. This book explores many of these factors and aims to position the general practitioner (GP) or allied health care practitioner (HCP) within modern day general practice to help make the best clinical decisions.

This book introduces many factors which GPs may take into account when consulting; some are rules and guidelines to improve practice and others are factors which we assimilate from our environments. External factors cannot be described without discussion of the consultation processes and the skills which GPs bring into consultations.

The clinical scenarios found in this book are both real and fictional. That is, they are derived from experience but none exist in the format described. The scenarios are common, the bread and butter of every day practice. Any identification with a real patient is totally coincidental. The end of each section signposts the reader to useful resources.

This book has been written with GP trainees and early year GPs in mind, and it should be useful for the MRCGP exam. This book is also relevant to HCPs who consult in primary care and any GP wanting an update. Whilst written within a general practice setting, this guide has relevance for all clinicians.

This book is not a textbook and is intended to be conversational in style. Will you be able to slot all illnesses and symptoms into easily accessed information systems by the end of this book? If this is your hope, stop right here, grab a cup of tea and come back! This book explores our reality; the ever-changing information we have at the time of decision making and the skills and difficulties doctors may have in accessing and applying these within the consultation. It is short, perhaps a two-day light read, but should be useful for years.

There are 4 main sections:

- Laws and regulations
- The consultation
- Knowledge and evidence
- Ethics and behaviours

At this point I want to let you know that I have specialised in general practice, that I love my job and that I love my patients. Love has many forms, and this is a professional love, a desire to help people through illness and uncertainty to live to their maximum potential. The bottom line is that we do our best for our patients and they appreciate it.

I hope you enjoy the read and have long and happy careers.

General Practice Today refers mainly to English law in general practice, and I refer to care givers as GPs, but information applies to other HCPs, GP trainees and clinical medical students.

There are a variety of consultation skill books, and I have enjoyed them all, but none more so than *The Inner Consultation* by Dr Roger Neighbour. I would like to acknowledge his contribution to the thinking of a generation of GPs. I do not offer a full synopsis of his book, a short discussion is within the consultation section, but I can recommend it to you as a good read. This book, *General Practice Today, a Practical Guide to Modern Consultations*, is mainly about all the other factors which sit with us when consulting.

Abbreviations

AA	Attendance Allowance
ACEI	Angiotensin Converting Enzyme Inhibitor
ACP	Advance Care Planning
ADRT	Advance Decision to Refuse Treatments
A&E	Accident and Emergency
AF	Atrial Fibrillation
AI	Artificial Intelligence
AMHP	Approved Mental Health Professional
AP	Assistant Practitioner
ARMD	Age Related Macular Degeneration
ARR	Absolute Risk Reduction
BCC	Basal Cell Cancer
BHF	British Heart Foundation
BNF	British National Formulary
BP	Blood Pressure
CCG	Clinical Commissioning Group
CHA_2DS_2VASc	a risk score used to calculate risk of systemic embolisation in atrial fibrillation
CHD	Coronary Heart Disease
COPD	Chronic Obstructive Pulmonary Disease
CPR	Cardiopulmonary Resuscitation
CTO	Community Treatment Order
CVA	Cerebrovascular Accident (stroke)
CXR	Chest X-ray
DAPT	Dual Antiplatelet Therapy
DBS	Disclosure and Barring Service
DLA	Disability Living Allowance
DNACPR	Do Not Attempt CPR
DSU	Drug Safety Unit
DVLA	Driver and Vehicle Licensing Authority
DVT	Deep Vein Thrombosis
ECG	Electrocardiogram
ECT	Electroconvulsive Therapy
eGFR	Electronic Glomerular Filtration Rate
e-LfH	e-Learning for Health
ENT	Ear, Nose and Throat

FBC	Full Blood Count
FGM	Female Genital Mutilation
FNeg	False Negative
FPA	Family Planning Association
FPos	False Positive
GMC	General Medical Council
GMS	General Medical Services
GP	General Practitioner
GTN	Glyceryl Trinitrate
HA	Health Assistant
HASBLED	a risk score used to calculate risk of bleeding on anticoagulants
HbA1c	Haemoglobin A1c
HBPM	Home Blood Pressure Monitoring
HCA	Health Care Assistant
HCP	Health Care Practitioner
HFEA	Human Fertilisation and Embryology Act
IBS	Irritable Bowel Syndrome
ICD	Implantable Cardioverter Defibrilator
IM	Intramuscular
IMB	Intermenstrual Bleeding
IMCAS	Independent Mental Capacity Advocate Service
IP	Inpatient
IT	Information Technology
IUCD	Intrauterine Contraceptive Device
IV	Intravenous
IVI	Intravenous Infusion
LPA	Lasting Power of Attorney
LN	Lymph Node
MCA	Mental Capacity Act
MDI	Metered Dose Inhaler
MDS	Monitored Dosage System
MEWS	Modified Early Waring Score
MHA	Mental Health Act
MI	Myocardial Infarction
mmHg	Millimetres of Mercury
MRI	Magnetic Resonance Imaging
MSF	Multisource Feedback
NEWS	National Early Warning Score
NHSE	National Health Service England
NICE	National Institute for Health and Care Excellence
NG	Nasogastric
NNT	Numbers Needed to Treat
NSC	National Screening Committee
OA	Osteoarthritis
od	Once Daily
OOH	Out of Hours

OPC	Outpatient Clinic
OTC	Over the Counter
PCME	Primary Care Medical Educators
PDA	Patient Decision Aids
PDP	Personal Development Plan
PE	Pulmonary Embolism
PEG	Percutaneous Gastroenterostomy
PGD	Patient Group Directions
PHE	Public Health England
PIL	Patient Information Leaflet
PIP	Personal Independence Payment
PMB	Postmenopausal
PMH	Past Medical History
PMR	Polymyalgia Rheumatic
PMS	Primary Medical Services
POM	Prescription Only Medication
PPAR	Peroxisome Proliferator-Activated Receptor
PPCI	Primary Percutaneous Coronary Angiography
PROMs	Patient Recorded Outcome Measures
PSD	Patient Specific Directions
PSQ	Patient Satisfaction Questionnaire
QoF	Quality and Outcomes Framework
RCGP	Royal College of General Practitioners
RCOG	Royal College of Obstetricians and Gynaecologists
SC	Subcutaneous
SIGN	Scottish Intercollegiate Guideline Network
SR	Sinus Rhythm
STI	Sexually Transmitted Infections
TIA	Transient Ischaemic Attack
T1IDDM	Type 1 Insulin Dependent Diabetic
T2DM	Type 2 Diabetic
TNeg	True Negative
TOP	Termination of Pregnancy
TPMT	Thiopurine Methyltransferase
TPos	True Positive Result
USS	Ultrasound Scan
2WW	2 Week Wait
WHO	World Health Organisation

Acknowledgments

This book would not have happened without the encouragement and help from lots of family, friends and colleagues. Also especially not without the wonderful patients I have been privileged to meet over the years. I would like to particularly thank Dr David Wilcock; David, my husband, who was my GP partner for 25 years at Silverdale (formerly Lowry) Medical Practice. David's love, thoughtfulness and support are simply without equal. Working with Dr Becky Holmes has been a joy and I cannot thank her enough for the work she has put into this book. Working with the illustrator, Grace Mutton, has been great fun and being able to ask colleagues and patients for their thoughts and views has been a privilege. I would also like to especially thank Selina Walsh for her excellent opinions throughout the writing of this book.

This book would also not have been possible without the exceptional skills of the publisher, Alice Oven. To have a publisher who, prior to having met me, offered excellent opinion, encouragement and loyalty is wonderful. I will always be grateful.

Those who have helped me with the preparation of this book, and who I would sincerely like to thank, are:

From Silverdale Medical Practice:

- Dr David Wilcock, MBChB, MRCGP, Cert.HE. Retired GP partner
- Mrs Andrea Simpson-Hague, AMSPAR. Practice manager
- Mrs Jackie Rivers, AMSPAR. Deputy Practice manager
- Dr Ian A. Ballin, MBChB, MRCGP, DRCOG, MEWI. GP senior partner
- Dr Zahid Ahmad, MBChB, DRCOG, Cert.GPEd. GP partner
- Dr Zehra Begum, MBBS, MRCGP, DFFP. GP partner

Mrs Selina Walsh, BSc (hons.), MSc advanced practice, MA, ethic care ethics and law, DPNS RN, RM. Advanced Nurse Practitioner and Registered Midwife, clinical ANP manager

Mrs Liz Smith, FDA, NVQ3 Health and Social care. Retired assistant practitioner.

Also all other staff and patients at Silverdale Medical Practice, Pendlebury Health Centre, Salford who have encouraged me and kept me on track.

Dr Sam Levinson, MBChB. Senior Partner Limefield Medical Practice, Salford

Mr Harvey Ward, BSc (hons. Econ), M.A, FRCGP (hon). Formerly lay chair of the RCGP's Patient and Carers Partnership Group. Current member of People in Partnership with the National Council for Palliative Care

Ms Nicola Wilcock, BSc (hons. theology) Dunelm

Ms Jennifer Wilcock, BA (hons. creative media)

Dr Ray Fewtrell, PhD. Director of Assessment, Lecturer in Medical Education, School of Medicine, Institute of Clinical Sciences, University of Liverpool for help with the Knowledge and evidence section.

Professor James McCormack, BSc (hons. Pharm), Pharm D, Professor Faculty of Pharmaceutical Sciences, UBC Vancouver, BC, Canada medicationmyth-busters.com for help with the knowledge and evidence section and for opening out conversations about evidence to thousands of doctors worldwide.

Dr Becky Holmes, MBChB Guardian Medical Centre, Warrington and community clinical tutor University of Liverpool School of Medicine

Dr Roger Neighbour, OBE MA DSc FRCGP FRCP FRACGP retired GP, former president RCGP, author of *The Inner Consultation, The Inner Apprentice* and *The Inner Physician* for his help with the synopsis of his *Inner Consultation* book.

Ms Grace Mutton, BA (hons. Illustration), illustrator. Contact email: gracemutton@gmail.com

Author Biography

Dr Jane Wilcock, BSc, FRCGP, PGCertMedEd, MAHEd, SFHEA, is an experienced GP. She graduated from Manchester University and has spent all her career, mostly full-time, in a practice in Salford, teaching undergraduates and as a postgraduate GP trainer. She held group teaching roles with the University of Manchester and was a primary care medical educator running a postgraduate GP trainee course for many years. More recently she has changed her primary role to facilitate medical education at the University of Liverpool School of Medicine and continues to work as a GP part-time.

Previous roles include GP trainer, PCME NW Deanery, undergraduate tutor in practice, group tutor for Manchester medical students, GP appraiser, curriculum year lead University of Liverpool School of Medicine and a past member of Greater Manchester, Lancashire and S. Cumbria Clinical Senate.

Currently, Dr Wilcock is a RCGP representative, a RCGP clinical advisor, a reviewer for Map of Medicine and NIHR projects. She is an undergraduate clinical tutor at the University of Liverpool and is also finals year assessment lead. In her free-time she is a GP author on update articles and medical education and a speaker for RCGP Mersey on womens health issues, for which she was awarded the 2015 Faculty award. She is an author of an online educational module for the RCOG and enjoys co-working with colleagues across universities.

She is interested in the use of information and is fascinated by the bombardment of health care workers with guidelines. She enjoys working as a part-time GP at the Silverdale Medical Practice where she has worked for 29 years, many of them with her husband. She enjoys talking to colleagues and patients about best care.

Laws and regulations

*In order to practice as the best doctors that we can be, we need to stop look-
ing over our shoulders like frightened children at laws that constrain us and
embrace them maturely as helpers to best practice. Lawmakers must ensure
there are as few laws as possible so that they are not overwhelming but are valued and practiced.*

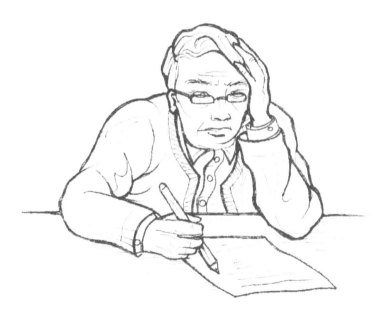

Hours of guidelines.

This section reviews some common legal duties that general practitioners (GPs)
should be aware of. There is a point at which 'those who decide for society' consider that an ethical position is so important that it must be enshrined in law. This
results in a number of recommendations for doctors to ensure they practice within

the law and supports them in their decisions. It also allows patients and their loved ones to have their wishes heard and hopefully met (more about this below). It can be a worry for busy doctors that they will fall foul of the law. This section highlights commonly met issues within English general practice, including the 3Cs – capacity, consent and confidentiality.

The information in this section is not exhaustive. This book is not a textbook of rules, nor does it cover all guidance. GPs work hard to offer care in the best interests of the patient but can run into circumstances that are difficult. Usually we find help and expertise amongst our practice teams, our defence bodies or occasionally through GMC advice. There is no discussion on the legal aspects of negligence and criminality – this book is a facilitator, not a frightener. Provided we practice with the patients' best interests as our focus and keep up to date, fear of negligence should not be a concern in our day-to-day practice.

Capacity and the Mental Capacity Act (MCA) 2005

In England and Wales, determining the patient's capacity is governed by the Mental Capacity Act (MCA) of 2005. In Scotland, it is the Adults with Incapacity Scotland Act 2000 and in N. Ireland there is no primary law. Here decision making for patients without capacity is governed by 'best interests' tests.

MCA DISCUSSION

People over 16 years old are assumed usually to have capacity and some children below 16 years old will also have capacity because of their intellectual maturity. GPs do not discriminate, particularly on grounds of age, in deciding whether someone has capacity; more about this later.

From the MCA:

1. *The following principles apply for the purposes of this Act.*
2. *A person must be assumed to have capacity unless it is established that he lacks capacity.*
3. *A person is not to be treated as unable to make a decision unless all practicable steps to help him to do so have been taken without success.*
4. *A person is not to be treated as unable to make a decision merely because he makes an unwise decision.*
5. *An act done, or decision made, under this Act for or on behalf of a person who lacks capacity must be done, or made, in his best interests.*
6. *Before the act is done or the decision is made, regard must be had to whether the purpose for which it is needed can be as effectively achieved in a way that is less restrictive of the person's rights and freedom of action.*

Capacity is easy to ascertain; after a bit of practice, it becomes second nature. GPs need to decide the following:

- Does the patient understand what is being said?
- Are they able to communicate their wishes to you clearly?

- Have they weighed up the pros and cons?
- Are they able to retain the information?

If there are difficulties with retention, then involving a friend, loved ones or other practice members (who know the patient) will help to make best decisions. Usually giving more time and written information helps. It is important that, unless in an absolute emergency, people are given every opportunity to understand and communicate their wishes. For example this may require translator services or changes in text size for someone with visual difficulty. Twelve per cent of those over the age of 80 have age-related macular degeneration and 2.5% of the over 50s.* Information about help that people need so that they can communicate and take in information should be highlighted on the patients' records and passed on to other agencies when needed.

Scenario: Poor vision and warfarin dosing
On receiving an outpatient clinic (OPC) letter from a cardiologist, a GP replied to the specialist to point out that the patient in question had poor vision and would have a lot of difficulty managing warfarin therapy, due to the variability in dosing over the week. In this case, a different anticoagulant with set dosing was preferable.

The Health and Social Care Act 2012 states that disabled people should have access to information they can understand and the communication support they may need. Therefore, ask patients and carers whether there is any help required. Implement this, record and highlight it. Share this information with others, if given permission by the patient.

Scenario: Transient lack of capacity in sepsis
Mr Y is 83 years old, usually self-caring and now unwell, in bed with wet bed sheets due to new onset urinary incontinence. His temperature is 38°C, pulse 100, sinus rhythm (SR) weak volume, blood pressure (BP) 110/70 mmHg. He takes amlodipine 5 mg od, ramipril 5 mg od, and occasionally a salbutamol metered dose inhaler (MDI). His chest is clear, abdomen soft and the GP makes a diagnosis of probable urinary sepsis and suggests hospital management. He refuses, saying, 'If I am to die, I want it to be here!'

His wife is not so sure he should stay at home.

The practical aspects of his care are that his BP is lower than usual, though he is rested in bed (his last three BP measurements have been around 136/84 mmHg according to his GP notes) and he hasn't eaten or drunk much for 24 hours. He needs his antihypertensive medication stopped. His pulse and temperature are consistent with sepsis. In addition, he requires blood tests to assess for acute kidney injury as he may have pre-renal failure from dehydration

---

* Owen CG, Jarrar Z, Wormald R, et al. The estimated prevalence and incidence of late stage age related macular degeneration in the UK. *British Journal of Ophthalmology* 2012;**96**:752–756.

with superadded ramipril-aggravated renal injury. On one hand, Mr Y might die, and being in his own home would be a preferable place for him with his wife in attendance; he is making that clear. But there is nothing in his scenario and pre-illness function to make the GP think that he will not make a good recovery with antibiotics. Antibiotics would preferably be intravenous initially in view of his sepsis. In this case, he needs clear information about his illness and the benefits and harms, including death, if he stays at home versus those if he is admitted. He can then weigh these options and decide whether to go into the hospital (which the GP and wife both feel to be the correct decision). If he has capacity, however, he is entitled to stay at home, if that is his wish. The GP should then manage him with blood tests, antibiotics, stopping antihypertensives and early review. In summary, people can make judgements that others disagree with if they have capacity to do so and this should be respected.

However, in this case Mr Y was agitated. He couldn't listen for long without interrupting and repeating himself. He couldn't relate what the benefits of hospital might be, even though they were explained so well that his wife was repeating them to him. He was unable to concentrate long enough to weigh up pros and cons of decisions and appeared unable to retain what was being said.

He therefore did not have capacity at that time. Professional guidance states that doctors should approach this man with the view of prolonging life if it is not clear that to do so would be futile and is not against any ADRT that he has made. The GP told him he was too unwell to decide on this occasion and arranged his admission. He came home pleased to have had treatment, with full recovery and had regained full cognition, reasoning and function.

Scenario: Communication issues
Mr Y had a severe stroke eight years ago and lives in a ground floor flat with regular carer visits. He has an expressive dysphasia, so he understands the spoken word but cannot use words to communicate his wishes reliably. He is able to say 'yes' and 'no' reliably though. He also has a visual field defect, so to see visitors they must stand to his right.

In order to take a history and test that he understands, his GPs only use questions which have a 'yes' or 'no' answer. His understanding is normal. When asked to put his right hand on his head, he will do so. When asked to do this with the left hand he tries but cannot, due to paralysis. Asked to say 'yes' or 'no' to whether he lives in Manchester, Leeds, London – this amused him – he can reply 'yes' for Manchester and 'no' for the others. Asked if he has a son and then if he has any daughters, he responds appropriately, confirming that he has a son but no daughters. He can therefore communicate and has capacity to understand. To communicate, the questioner should be creative about the type of questions asked. So, a GP would not ask, 'How long have you felt ill?' but might ask, 'Have you been ill more than one day?', 'more than one week?', etc. The question 'where is the pain?' is inappropriate but 'do you have any pain?' is a reliable question for him. In this way, the history can be narrowed down.

Scenario: Another communication issues

Mr Y communicates only by eye movements. He has no speech at all but can communicate by deviating his eyes up or down reliably to mean 'yes' and 'no'.

Again, the GP should check capacity and ask a history in a way which allows the patient to communicate effectively. These histories take time and patience but are very rewarding.

Having a mental illness does not necessarily mean a patient lacks capacity. Of course, if a patient is psychotic then they may not have capacity, as they may have disordered thoughts. This is especially true in acute psychotic episodes. However, many patients have a diagnosis of psychosis on their records but have become well enough to have capacity, live independently and make informed choices. A GP should therefore be careful to avoid prejudice in deciding capacity based on someone's past medical history.

FRASER GUIDELINES FOR CONTRACEPTION PROVISION IN THE UNDER 16s

Sex is illegal for boys and girls under 16 years old. Under 13 years old, sex is rape. Of course, there are young people who fall in love and decide to have sex but may not yet be 16 years old. There may be no concerns about grooming, abuse, etc. They may attend to ask for emergency contraception, to discuss future contraception or to start it when already sexually active. GPs can provide contraception to under 16 year olds if they believe it is in the young person's best medical interests, if the young person is able to give informed consent, and if they have tried to persuade the young person to talk about contraception with their parent or other trusted adult. To consent the young person must have capacity.

In 1986 Mrs Gillick (Gillick v West Norfolk and Wisbech AHA 1986) complained that she should have been informed and asked for consent when her daughter, under 16 years old, was prescribed contraception. From this case, in deciding whether the young person can have contraception provided, Lord Fraser developed guidelines* which unsurprisingly state that the GP needs to be satisfied on a number of key issues:

The doctor will, in my opinion, be justified in proceeding without the parents' consent or even knowledge provided he is satisfied on the following matters:

1. *That the girl (although under 16 years of age) will understand his advice*
2. *That he cannot persuade her to inform her parents or to allow him to inform the parents that she is seeking contraceptive advice*
3. *That she is very likely to begin or to continue having sexual intercourse with or without contraceptive treatment*
4. *That unless she receives contraceptive advice or treatment her physical or mental health or both are likely to suffer*

---

* e-law resources including about the Fraser guidelines at: http://www.e-lawresources. co.uk/cases/Gillick-v-West-Norfolk.php.

5. *That her best interests require him to give the contraceptive advice, treatment or both without the parental consent.*

Outcomes of pregnancy in the under 16s can be poor; many result in abortion and mental upset. Those who continue with pregnancy have increased hazards in pregnancy, e.g. eclampsia and an increased risk of perinatal death. The girl's future life is changed dramatically and often the grandparents of the baby too.

Scenario: Contraception request from a 15-year-old girl

Miss X, 15 years old, attends the GP because she had sex with her long-term boyfriend the night before and then told her friends. They told her to attend the GP for the 'morning after pill' in case she gets pregnant. So, she has come in after school. She is in the middle of her menstrual cycle.

This girl has already had sex and the GP needs to approach this with a logical sequence. The doctor should fulfil the Fraser guidelines, asking whether her parents or guardians know she is having sex and whether she can talk to them about it. If not there may be another adult, like an aunt or grandparent, who she could confide in. If not, enquire why not. She may let the GP inform her parents rather than doing it herself.

If she had not had unprotected sex but was looking to start contraception, the GP might opt to ask her to return with a parent. In the scenario above though, the girl was not willing to tell anyone in her family. She was mature enough to know what she was doing but felt her parents would not approve and did not want to confide in anyone, except her friends. The GP established that she had capacity to understand contraceptive information.

The GP should also consider whether the relationship may be abusive. In this instance, her 'long-term relationship' meant she had been seeing a boy in her class for three months and that they were both in love. He was 'the one!' The GP had uncovered that this was not an abusive relationship but a consensual act.

The GP should talk about the risks of sexually transmitted infections (STIs), recommend infection screening immediately (and in 2 weeks for chlamydia incubation), and promote and offer condoms. It is remarkable that condoms are not on GP prescription pads! There are schemes providing condoms in some practices but not for all age groups. The GP should talk about the girl's periods, eliciting whether this was the first episode of sex this cycle, and considering risks of pre-existing pregnancy. At this point the GP should discuss and offer emergency contraception, which might be the copper coil (and probably azithromycin 1G at insertion in case of chlamydial infection), levonorgestrel, e.g. Levonelle, or ulipristal (UPA), e.g. ellaOne, and discuss or provide on-going contraception. The girl should be given family planning association literature (or provided with the web address if more likely to use the Internet than read a leaflet). The GP should arrange review and arrange a pregnancy test three weeks later if she has not had her usual period. There is a lot to this simple request and, as always, good record keeping is mandatory.

Consent

This second area in the Laws and Regulations section discusses the types of consent commonly found in general practice.

Most of the time, GP consent requires a patient with capacity to be given enough information to be able to make good judgements for themselves, with the support of their doctor. Usually verbal, it may be written or may just be implied. Anyone 16 years old or older is presumed to have capacity to consent but the under 16s should be involved in discussions about preference, with some being mature enough to consent for themselves. Written consent is usual if the possible complications of the decision may be serious. Consent should be recorded in the notes and it is helpful to state whether written material has been given. Doctors are required to follow GMC guidance and should work within their limits: if put on the spot over an item which you are not expert in, defer the decision and talk to your colleagues.

Consent requires the GP and patient to discuss the condition using all the information available at the time. The GP also discusses the risks and benefits, and lets the patient know how to proceed, often with reasonable options, but suggesting their best practice recommendation for that patient at that time, and using language that the patient understands. Some patients do not want their doctor to give preferences and this should be respected, but most people want to have expert guidance with control over the final decision left to themselves. The GP listens whilst the patient weighs up the options, benefits and risks and opts for a course of action. The GP should explore the patient's decision further if it is surprising and they disagree with it; but if the patient is sure and has capacity, then their wishes should ultimately be followed. If the patient appears not to have capacity then the GP should work with the patient's loved ones and the primary care team to make the best decision for that person. The decision should be recorded accurately in the notes. The GP needs to avoid jargon and use plain English or use confidential translating services, not family members, to ensure communication is optimal.

Scenario: Example of jargon
Mr Y is 67 years old and attends the GP, 'I have come this afternoon, doctor, because the chest specialist this morning said I had a tumour. I want to know, does that mean I have a cancer?'

Scenario: Wanting expert advice
Mrs X is 80 years old and has been diagnosed with cancer. She attends the GP, 'I have come to see you, doctor, because the specialist said I could have radiotherapy or surgery or chemotherapy and I don't know which one to choose. When I asked him, he said it was up to me to decide'.

This type of cancer is always best treated with surgery if possible but this fact had not been given to the patient – just the options.

IMPLIED CONSENT

Implied consent is used when material harm is unlikely to result to a patient with capacity and in which he/she attends or does something (like rolling up a sleeve) with the procedure in mind to show assent.

Scenario: BP check

Mrs X is 60 years old and takes an antihypertensive drug, amlodipine 5 mg once a day. She attends the GP practice for a BP check with the assistant practitioner (AP). She sits in the chair, takes off her coat and rolls her sleeve up.

This is implied consent because she knows why she has attended and is preparing for the test. She does not need detailed counselling.

Is that it then? Well, it follows GMC guidance but in a professional sense we can do better. The excellent health care practitioner (HPC) would let her know her BP reading (preferably written down so that she can share the information with family, friends and sometimes OPC, accurately). She needs to know her BP result, her expected BP target and whether she meets this. In this way, she is aware of her own blood pressure control, is more likely to adhere to lifestyle and therapy plans and understands the need for treatment modification if required. Asking about medication side-effects would be outside of an APs knowledge base but would be a GP function.

Of course, if she has been previously counselled and has this information already, then her action is truly implied consent.

Scenario: Cholesterol check because of family bereavement

Mr Y is 45 years old and attends for a well-person check with the AP. He asks for a cholesterol check because his mother died recently, at 76 years old, of a sudden heart attack. He rolls up his sleeve.

This is implied consent for venepuncture and does not require a detailed consent discussion of law in order to have the test. However, the excellent HCP would point out that mother's heart attack at 76 years old, with no other family history, is not premature and may represent a natural end to a life. The patient should still have counselling about a healthy lifestyle to prevent heart disease and after venepuncture be told how and when to receive information about the result. *Is this enough?* In addition, the patient requires information about the level of cholesterol which would be enough to recommend statin therapy if he is found to have primary (familial) hypercholesterolaemia. He should be asked whether he wants a risk score to decide whether his lifestyle, age, male sex, etc. combined with the result would initiate a suggestion of statin therapy.

So, there are no easy answers if patients are to receive modern health care and no easy, short appointments. Unfortunately, due to time pressures, much of this is not routinely done initially and the patient too often returns to a confusing, piecemeal programme of poor or partial information, recalls, rechecks and confusion.

Scenario: Venepuncture for sore throat

Mr Y, 27 years old, attends with a sore throat. He came a week ago but his throat is just as sore and he is off his food, living on soup for a week, and feels drained.

A week previously a GP wrote:

Four days of worsening sore throat; eating OK. No cough, tender neck, no rash, feels hot. Exam: temp 37.8° C, pulse 88 SR, BP 120/70 mmHg. Tender 0.5 cm lymph nodes (LNs) × 3 neck, chest clear, neck flexion good, no rash, white exudate both tonsils, airway fair.

Diagnosis Tonsillitis, likely bacterial

Plan: no PMH, no drug allergies; treat penicillin V (phenoxymethylpenicillin 500 mg × 4 a day for 5 days) see if problems.

Today the GP finds the signs are unchanged despite the patient finishing a five-day course of phenoxymethylpenicillin. Our GP thinks this course is a little short and wonders about a throat swab, but suggests first to take the patient's blood to test for glandular fever (Epstein Barr virus, infectious mononucleosis) and the patient starts to roll up his sleeve. This is implied consent. Nevertheless, discussion about why the blood test is being done, i.e. a test for glandular fever but also a check on neutrophilia (as neutrophilia indicates a bacterial infection) and consideration of liver enzymes to look for an associated viral hepatitis, does require a short explanation.

You may realise by this point that I really don't much like implied consent! It may lower standards and encourages GPs to miss opportunities to get the basics right and educate the patient. Governments need to recognise professionalism and facilitate longer consulting times, to save time in the long run and optimise health care.

CONSENT IN AN ADULT WITH CAPACITY

GPs, for the most part, are not burdened with the terrible consequences of procedures that our secondary care colleagues may unfortunately bear during their career. For surgeons in particular, consent is a detailed and laborious process designed to ensure patient understanding and improve safety.

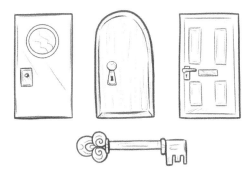

One key doesn't open all doors...

Nonetheless, for GPs there are many times when consent in an adult with capacity is important. It might be a steroid injection into a joint or tendon sheath, performing a vaginal examination and swabs, discussion of appropriate therapeutic options, suggesting hospital admission or removing a sebaceous cyst. The rule to remember is to consider not what a reasonable doctor might think, but what a reasonable patient might expect to know. This includes risks, benefits and management options and includes the doctor's preferred option – it does not negate our responsibility to offer best medical advice at the time, even if this is not subsequently selected by the patient. Consent must be voluntary, by a patient with capacity, and informed.

In 2015, consent was improved by the case of *Montgomery (Appellant) v Lanarkshire Health Board (Respondent)*.* The case revolved around information-giving. In 1999, a patient with diabetes was not told of the risks of shoulder dystocia in vaginal delivery because her obstetrician had decided that it was in the patient's best interests to have a vaginal birth. Unfortunately, there were awful difficulties. The baby got stuck in the birth canal with a difficult shoulder dystocia, resulting in birth injury to the baby, traumatic delivery for the mum, and a completely unexpected outcome for the family for years to come due to looking after a child with severe disability. Like almost all 'accidents', in hindsight, things could have been improved and done differently. The main issue though, was that the mum felt that the risks of dystocia, which were estimated at about 10%, should have been discussed with her and an opportunity to discuss methods of birth made available. The judgement agreed and made it clear that the risk was not about percentage risk but about the individual's perception of risk to them as individuals.

This had been explored in Australia in the 1993 case of *Rogers v Whitaker*. A man who only had vision in one eye had a procedure on the other which led to an unusual complication and subsequent blindness. The complication was so unusual that it was not usual practice for the ophthalmic surgeon to mention it to his patients. The patient stated that had he been aware of the risk, being uni-ocular, he would have weighed this up in advance before agreeing to the operation on his seeing eye.

The law states that judgements should depend on what a reasonable patient would think and do in those circumstances.

The GMC guidance on consent starts with *Good Medical Practice* and suggests consent should relate to examinations, investigations, treatments, teaching and research; though it should include any aspect of medical care including history taking, as illustrated below. It is expanded in the GMC guidance, *Consent: doctors and patients making decisions together,* which starts with *Duties of a Doctor.* The first and perhaps the only guidance needed for any GP is

'Make the care of your patients your first concern'.

* Judgement Montgomery (Appellant) v Lanarkshire Health Board (Respondent) (Scotland) The Supreme Court UK at https://www.supremecourt.uk/decided-cases/docs/UKSC_2013_0136_Judgment.pdf.

Consent should not be about a tick box form which covers all eventualities and should not offer so much intricate detail that the patient cannot understand it. GPs try to remember a plethora of medical knowledge so having some accurate written literature to remind us, and our patients, about risks and benefits is invaluable. Indeed, having some accurate literature to give to patients to think about, if the consent is not urgent, allows them to reflect on the information, discuss it with family and friends if they want to, and make better decisions. The principle of patient autonomy firmly lays the doctor's traditional and outdated desire for paternalism to bed. In an age when almost all adults can read and many, of all ages, are adept at skilling up on the Internet, the shift to enablement has arrived.

Scenario: Patient doesn't want information

Mr Y attends for his first post-operative prescription for his colostomy bags. He relates to his GP that when being consented for the op the consultant started to 'go on about loads of things that could go wrong in the operation. I told him I didn't want to hear that, just give me the paper and let me sign. I knew I had a colon cancer and I wouldn't have gone in for the op if I didn't trust him would I?'

Mr Y is completely rational, does not want a lot of information and trusts his surgeon. He can sign the consent form without having to hear a lot of detail and his consultant should record that. Some patients do not want to be told all the pros and cons of a procedure and do not have to be forced to hear it. They do, however, have to show capacity.

Scenario: Consent is scenario specific

Miss X, 24 years old, attends with a cough. An older woman, clearly her mum, comes in with her. The GP checks it is her mum and asks whether it is alright to have her mum present. Miss X consents to her mum being present.

At the end of the conversation Miss X says, 'Whilst I'm here can I have my usual contraception, Microgynon30, to save me coming back?' The GP gets the prescription upon the repeat prescription screen and asks, 'Are you having any problems with it?' to which this scenario plays out:

Miss X: 'No, I think it is good, but I am getting some bleeding in the middle of my cycle a few times, is that usual?'

You will recognise now that the GP needs to take a detailed gynaecological and sexual history. It may cause a sigh as time is ticking on and the GP had assumed it was a quick request, but the patient has now opened a whole new consultation. But about consent:

GP: 'I want to ask you some personal questions which may be relevant to the bleeding. Do you still want your mum in?'
Miss X: 'Yes I tell her everything, we're really close!'
GP progressively asks: 'How long have you had the bleeding, how long does it last, do you have a partner, do you have sex?'

At this point, Miss X glances at her mum, looks embarrassed, and hesitates. The GP picks up the cue.

GP: *'We could ask your mum to wait outside whilst I ask the personal questions, if you like?'*

Miss X nods and mum looks relieved to escape into the waiting area.

It transpires that Miss X has a rocky relationship with her boyfriend and they have recently 'made up' again after a hiatus in the relationship. She also has some new vaginal discharge. There are some things you don't want your mum to know!

This scenario is fairly common in primary care and illustrates that consent is specific to the circumstances and changeable. Doctors should keep on their mental toes and think ahead.

Scenario: Consent does not mean giving too much technical information (how much is too much?)
Thank you to the patient who consented to including this in the book. Mrs X has been through diagnosis and management of breast cancer and has been offered breast reconstruction. She wants this and comes to see the GP with her OPC letter. The letter details the procedure in order to allow her to have informed consent.

Mrs X: *'What do you think of this, doctor, it is very scary? I don't really understand it. Should I go ahead?'*

Parts of the letter are below:
As we discussed, it is a microsurgical operation, which can take 8–10 hours and occasionally can last longer if there are any intraoperative issues that require attention. It involves removing the skin and fat from the lower abdominal wall based on the blood supply from the deep inferior epigastric artery perforator. This is then transposed to the chest wall and the blood vessels are joined up under a microscope to the blood vessels in the chest, which we can access by removing a small piece of cartilage connecting the rib to the sternum. You will have a scar...
We will also have to introduce a paddle of tummy skin to your breasts...
We also discussed the risks of surgery, which is a microscopic procedure and has a 2–5% failure rate. There is a risk of some fat necrosis in the reconstructed breasts and occasionally delayed wound healing. In the abdomen, these same risks apply....
You could experience seroma, delayed wound healing, and numbness round the scar, as well as general risks from a big operation such as deep vein thrombosis and pulmonary embolus.
Secondary revision surgery is usually required....
We will organise a CT angiogram, to look at the blood vessels of the tummy wall....
I hope this has been helpful to you and if you have any questions please write them down and bring them with you when you come back to see me again.....

This is a clear, well-communicated letter, although rates of DVT or other serious complications could have been included. However, the patient had been getting panic disorder since reading it and backtracked on her desire to have the operation. It was too much for her to take in. There is a difference between taking information in for yourself and being a patient. In this case, the GP had a detailed consultation which settled her mind and let her make her own decision, not swayed by panic at the technical jargon she had read.

EMERGENCIES AND CONSENT

If an emergency arose and the doctor can't possibly know the patient's wishes, then the GP should act and treat the patient without their consent to save their life or to prevent a serious deterioration in their condition. Once the patient can consent, or perhaps relatives arrive with further information or advance decisions, then consent and capacity may become clearer and treatment decisions can be reviewed to match the patient's best interests and wishes.

There is no legal obligation for doctors to stop and help in an emergency in England. However, most of us would if we felt we could contribute helpfully. Most GPs are not skilled first responders though, and it is therefore up to the individual GP. Many GPs have stopped at accidents until the ambulance has arrived but, as always in medicine, it would depend upon the circumstances. Doctors who have recently done an accident and emergency (A&E) hospital post are very different to those who have not done any emergency care for 25 years.

Useful resources for consent and capacity:

- Mental capacity act 2005 at: http://www.legislation.gov.uk/ukpga/2005/9/contents
- GMC Good Medical Practice at http://www.gmc-uk.org/guidance/good_medical_practice.asp
- GMC Consent: patients and doctors making decisions together at: http://www.gmc-uk.org/guidance/ethical_guidance/consent_guidance_index.asp
- NSPCC site on Fraser guidelines at: https://www.nspcc.org.uk/preventing-abuse/child-protection-system/legal-definition-child-rights-law/gillick-competency-fraser-guidelines/

Difficult decisions: Legal frameworks and guidelines in end of life care

End of life guidelines is a difficult area for GPs and requires some endurance of the guidance for practitioners to catch up and become used to the difficulties and details of decision making for patients. It is also a new and strange area for the patient and their loved ones to navigate (not because people haven't always ultimately died) but because the guidance has now become formalised. Hopefully the summaries below and resources at the end of the section will not only help us make best decisions and follow the latest guidance, but also retain an overview of this topic as other health care team members take on specific roles. In this way, we can be confident that care is always in the best interests of our patients.

It is an accepted definition that the end of life relates to the stage in which people with ill health are not expected to live for more than 12 months. This is helpful for patients with degenerative conditions, e.g. most motor neurone diseases or aggressive terminal cancers in which the clinical picture usually follows a recognised downward pattern. However, many patients with 'terminal' diagnoses defy the odds and live good quality lives within the framework of their disability, sometimes astounding their doctors for many years. There are also enormous numbers of elderly people with dementia and it is common to live 10 years with this condition, despite the individuals starting their journey to the end of life at the start of their diagnosis. Other people develop frailty and lots of current research looks at definitions of frailty and encourages clinicians to consider the patient's holistic function across medical, social, physical and psychological areas of their lives. GPs who have had continuity of care for their population over decades are best placed to recognise changes and end of life proximity. However, the modern NHS has removed (deconstructed) much role continuity, replacing this with recommendations and guidance to create uniform working practices. In English general practice, the quality and outcomes framework (QoF), a part of the GPs' contract to provide care states:

Records PC001. The contractor establishes and maintains a register of all patients in need of palliative care/support irrespective of age.

Ongoing management PC002. The contractor has regular (at least three monthly) multidisciplinary case review meetings where all patients on the palliative care register are discussed.

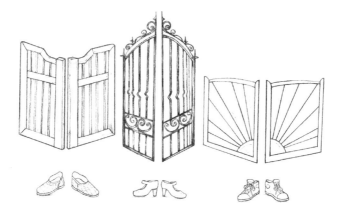

We open many different gates and journey down different paths in our lives but we don't all travel the same journey and even if we do, we may not be wearing the same shoes.

This provides a framework to coordinate the patient's views and those of the health care team and improve care for those expected to die. At present, most patients will die in hospital but would prefer to die at home. This can be difficult as nursing care can become continuous, day and night, for some in the end stages of life; even recognising dying can be difficult and variable. However, a lot of excellent work has gone into helping GPs and their teams provide good quality end of life care for people in their own homes. As the QoF document states, *'A quarter of all deaths are due to cancer, a third from organ failure, a third from frailty or dementia and only one twelfth of patients have a sudden death. It may therefore be possible to predict the majority of deaths, however, this is difficult and errors occur 30 per cent of the time. Two thirds of errors are based on over optimism and one third on pessimism'.*

Patients at the end of life may require financial help and the general practice team, McMillan support nurses, social workers, or other health care workers can recommend that the patient collects a disability living allowance (DLA) or attendance allowance (AA) and that their carer may qualify for a carers allowance. DLA is being replaced by personal independence payments (PIPs) during 2017. The patient who is likely to die in the next 12 months can have the claim fast-tracked by issuing a DS1500 'special rules' form by the GP. The patient may require information about other services like a disabled parking badge and it is the GPs role to help coordinate teams, including out-of-hours (OOH) care, to provide best care and access to appropriate services.

Patients may or may not have capacity to make decisions or they may be in a position of being able to make decisions now, but understand that this is likely to vanish as their disease progresses. They may want to make a will or think about their funeral. If they have capacity, they may want to nominate a Lasting Power of Attorney (see below). We must use clear plain language and may need to provide translators, written material, time and revisiting their problems to allow best decisions from our patients, maximising their ability to be involved. GPs should ensure good communication with other health and social care providers who might be important to decisions and care. Disputes in care may require second opinions.

Although we like to be concordant with wishes of family and friends, illness is hard to bear and fall-outs and disputes may occur within families. Sometimes GPs receive conflicting wishes from different family members. To create fairness and clarity there are several legal obligations stated in the MCA, 2005. If there is a dispute this may be resolved informally, by the practice complaints procedure, or the complainant may take legal action. Therefore, good record keeping about decisions and management plans is important. In general, though, exploration of the issues should resolve most problems. Patients with capacity always have an ability to make up their own minds, regardless of family and friend views. If a GP is in a position in which he/she feels that the treatment a patient wants is not reasonable and can justify this, the GP does not have to provide it. We must work with our patients but we must also respect our professional values and knowledge. Most patients appreciate the help we give but there are unpleasant and difficult people the world through, and having open access as GPs we and our teams will meet them, and it will be difficult. Finding a patient or relative difficult, aggressive or bullying is not a professional reason to acquiesce to a demand which is unreasonable. GPs must however be able to justify their decisions. When in doubt seek help from team members and second opinions. Fortunately, although memorable, difficulties are unusual.

For patients who are alone and lack capacity, they are supported by the independent mental capacity advocate service (IMCAS). This service offers support and will act to represent the patient's interests.

In general, GMC guidance states that if there is uncertainty about the benefits of therapy, treatment should be started with advance discussion about how it will be monitored, why, and when it might be withdrawn. The onus is on prolonging life if there is doubt. Any decision can be changed, if justified, when the patient's circumstances change.

Patients near the end of life should have reviews of their hydration and nutrition status and a decision made about their requirements, i.e. what is required as food and fluid for the individual. It may be that the patient requires clinically assisted nutrition, e.g. by nasogastric (NG) tube, percutaneous gastroenterostomy (PEG), which is a tube through the skin into the stomach, intravenous infusion (IVI), or subcutaneous (SC) infusion of fluids. Commencing this is usually done in secondary care. If commenced in primary care this requires a discussion with the practice team. It should be started if clinically indicated and wanted by the patient or decision maker. Withdrawing and withholding nutrition and fluids is difficult. It might be very inappropriate in the end days or hours of life to be technically introducing equipment, fluids and nutrition but if the patient has made it clear that they want this, then their wishes will usually be respected.

Scenario: Excellent carers
It was an unusually hot day, during a heat wave and the tiniest, oldest, most infirm lady in the practice was looked after by carers three times a day. She must have had the practice's greatest frailty index! Her GP dropped by (the elderly neighbour had a key,) concerned that she might be overheated or dry. Her carers had kept the curtains closed where the sun shone through and had sat longer than usual with her over meals and recorded her fluid intake. She told the GP, 'They are fantastic you know'. They had left her a big drink of orange squash within reach too.

Fantastic carers.

Some patients, aware they may lose capacity, make their loved and trusted ones attorneys for their care. This is discussed next.

LASTING POWER OF ATTORNEY (LPAs)
This is outlined in law in the Mental Capacity Act of 2005.

Scenario: Early dementia

Mr Y, 84 years old, has become increasingly forgetful. His daughter, 58 years old, has taken to doing his shopping and popping in after work each day to ensure he has a meal. He pays her the shopping bill money directly. He has always paid his other bills but now she sees that his mail is left unopened and she is anxious about this. After a sleepless night one day she guiltily opens his mail and finds that he has not paid his gas bill. She confronts him with the problem and he agrees that he is getting a bit forgetful and that she should manage his bills from now on. He agrees that she can access his bank account, as they have a trusting relationship. She speaks to a solicitor by phone and makes an appointment to bring her dad into the solicitor's office. He and she are counselled by the solicitor and her dad is pleased to sign for her to be the Lasting Power of Attorney (LPA) for property and affairs. The daughter ensures that he can live comfortably at home and she is not anxious about his finances and bills any more.

Lots of families and friends pay bills for their loved ones and keep them informally safe. Problems occur when the patient can't remember their passwords or numbers to access their money to pay for their shopping or cease to be bothered by bills! Knowing that was likely to become a bigger issue in the example above, the daughter decided to implement an LPA for Property and Affairs – there is also a Personal Welfare LPA.

Property and Affairs LPA: this is for people who can make decisions (have capacity) and for those without capacity and allows the designated Attorney to make decisions about financial matters

Personal Welfare LPA: this is for people who cannot make decisions (lack capacity) to allow the designated Attorney to make decisions, knowing the patient's views on care, including end of life care and life-sustaining treatment, etc.

They can be revoked legally if misused.

ADVANCE STATEMENTS AND ADVANCE CARE PLANNING (ACP)

Anyone can say or write down what they would like to happen if they become unable to state them at the time of illness. An advance statement sets out the person's preferences for care. Written statements are more compelling and provable than remembered verbal statements. They will be considered but are not legally binding if thought not to be in the best interests of the patient.

Scenario: Advance care plan (ACP)

Mrs X has been diagnosed with Huntington's chorea and is currently well with some chorea-type movements. She writes an advanced care plan on a notepad and gives it to the GP. The GP asks her to record it on an Advanced Care Plan template but stresses that she doesn't have to use the proforma and creates a scanned copy of the ACP from the patient's notebook to sit in her records. The GP tells Mrs X that she can change her mind at any time but to let the practice know if this happens.

Mrs X goes home to complete the form as she liked the template and will keep it somewhere safe. What had she written? She has stated a wish that her older sister make decisions for her if she is unable. Also, that she be looked after in a local care home if incapable of managing self-care. The reason for this was that her sister had had a bad accident and walked with two crutches, so she wanted professional help rather than family help. She had no views about what happened once she had died.

So, wishes can be formalised into an ACP. For the patient above, the GP would try to acquiesce to her wishes and is aware of the rationale behind them. An ACP is not legally binding and if she can be kept at home without her sister being involved in personal care the practice would facilitate this. The patient understands this but the practice has now acknowledged that it might be that a care or nursing home would be a better choice if her sister was expecting to act as carer.

ACPs are a developing area and entail formally recording discussions with the patients (of any age) to determine their wishes about therapy and care. An ACP is normally used for people at the end of life but can be used earlier and allows them to talk through likely future choices and provides a record of wishes in case they do lose the capacity to make themselves understood. In effect, discussions are recorded, decisions about who can know the information agreed upon, and the document becomes a future care plan. It is voluntary. Some people do not like to think about death and dying and cope much better without this conversation, but for others it is very useful. There is a move to have shared online sites for patients, e.g. Coordinate My Care was developed in London in 2012 to create an online record for urgent care for patients so that out of hours (OOH) services, GPs, secondary care, and the patient him/herself can access the care plan in real time.

The GMC guidance states that ACP discussions should include the following:

If a patient in your care has a condition that will impair their capacity as it progresses, or is otherwise facing a situation in which loss or impairment of capacity is a foreseeable possibility, you should encourage them to think about what they might want for themselves should this happen, and to discuss their wishes and concerns with you and the health care team. Your discussions should cover:

1. *The patient's wishes, preferences or fears in relation to their future treatment and care. Feelings, beliefs or values that may be influencing the patient's preferences and decisions*
2. *The family members, others close to the patient or any legal proxies that the patient would like to be involved in decisions about their care*
3. *Interventions which may be considered or undertaken in an emergency, such as cardiopulmonary resuscitation (CPR), when it may be helpful to make decisions in advance*
4. *The patient's preferred place of care (and how this may affect the treatment options available) and for some letting health carers know about after-death preparations.*

ADVANCE DECISIONS TO REFUSE TREATMENT (ADRT)

Advance decisions to refuse treatment are written statements which are signed and witnessed, and have a specific statement saying that the advance decision is applied even if the patient's life is at risk. They normally pertain to refusing life sustaining treatment. They are legally binding for all including the GP, practice team, and relatives. The individual must have capacity when creating an ADRT and the instructions should be specific. If the document is not legally binding then it should still be considered; it carries less legal weight, though may still accurately reflect the patient's views. Be careful to make records as patients with capacity can withdraw their decisions if they wish. If there is an emergency and you are uncertain of the patient's wishes, or if any ADRT is made, then you should act to prolong life until the situation is clearer.

Scenario: ADRT

Mr Y has lung cancer and refuses hospitalisation because his wife and his two sisters have died in hospital and he has a morbid fear of them. He has decided that if his lung cancer deteriorates he would not want chemotherapy, radio-therapy, artificial feeding or antibiotics, even if he had a chest infection. He has written this down and his friend, who has come to see the GP with him, has signed it as a witness. The GP checks that, with his consent, he/she can share this with the secondary care services and the district nursing team. Being organised, the patient had already done this but wanted to meet his GP to let him/her know.

If you cannot agree with a patient's decision on religious or moral grounds then you will need to find another GP or HCP to take over the care of that patient.

DO NOT ATTEMPT CARDIOPULMONARY RESUSCITATION (DNACPR)

As a newly qualified hospital doctor, many of us have responded to an emer-gency resuscitation bleep in hospitals and run to a bedside to try to resuscitate someone who clearly had illnesses which were not reversible by cardiopulmo-nary resuscitation (CPR). Resuscitation can be effective for some acute problems and the main one is ventricular fibrillation. Doctors have long wondered why people weren't asked if they wanted resuscitation on admission to hospital. In general practice some years ago, a terminally ill patient, who had died a few hours before and had regular GP visits, had CPR. The GP had told the wife that she didn't need to call the ambulance if he died but she did as she understand-ably panicked. Later, she vividly described the emergency efforts at CPR which were traumatic and futile. She regretted the 999 call. A DNACPR form would have informed the ambulance service that CPR was not required and that this was an expected death.

Recently a patient related how she rushed to the hospital after her elderly demented mum had fallen badly at home. On the ward, the consultant approached waving a DNACPR form and it was the first item the specialist mentioned. She was traumatised by the experience, as there was no introduction or discussion to the topic; it was tactless. Patients with capacity have a right to be a part of the discussion and some will want to decide to refuse CPR or not. The doctor should have a discussion with the patient and next of kin (if the patient agrees) about DNACPR and record this in the notes on a DNACPR form.

If the patient lacks capacity, their personal welfare LPA should be asked (if there is one). If there is no personal welfare LPA then their carer or loved ones should be consulted. The names and relationships of those involved in the discussion should be recorded in line with good record keeping. The patient with no-one to represent their wishes should have an IMCA appointed and consulted. The DNACPR decision should be reviewed at stated intervals and the decision communicated to those who are a part of the health care team. Ambulance and OOH services also need to be informed about this decision.

In general, the patient's request will be honoured but if GPs feel it is not in the patient's best interests to be resuscitated, and can justify this, they can make the final decision. However, it would be wise in a dispute to seek a second opinion.

IMPLANTABLE CARDIOVERTER DEFIBRILLATOR (ICD) DEACTIVATION

Discussing deactivation of an implanted defibrillator is a difficult, unpleasant topic. A patient maintained in good health through technology may find it becomes uncomfortable at the end of life. This sort of scenario will become more common with technological advances.

Scenario: ICD deactivation

Miss X, 50 years old, has an advanced pancreatic cancer. She is in the last days of life, in bed, jaundiced, and feels lethargic. She was fitted with an ICD about 10 years ago after two episodes of collapse. She was found to have episodes of ventricular tachycardia and has not had a collapse since the ICD was fitted.

This patient is at risk of her ICD giving her unpleasant electric shocks as she dies. After death, movement of the body may cause inappropriate electrical shocks which family, funeral services or HCPs might feel and may cause distress. The doctor should discuss the issue with the patient and, if he/she agrees, fill in a deactivation form and arrange an appointment with the programmer or a house visit by the programmer to deactivate the ICD. In emergency situations, e.g. not having a programmer available, GPs may be advised to collect a magnet from the cardiology department which, when positioned over the ICD, deactivates it. The next of kin should be involved in the decision if possible. The device can be reactivated if the patient's condition improves. If there is disagreement between yourself and the patient or carer, then gain a second opinion from the palliative care specialist team. The British Heart Foundation (BHF) does mention the issue of deactivation in their patient guide to ICDs, which is given during the fitting.

PALLIATIVE THERAPY

Patients requiring palliative care require skilled GPs and teams. There are excellent resources from palliative care specialists and one in the resources below. This details emergency cancer care problems, e.g. hypercalcaemia and spinal cord compression, and also prescribing in end of life care and use of syringe drivers. The British National Formulary (BNF) and eBNF also have excellent palliative care sections, including tables of equivalence for different types of opiate and doses. Using this guide clinicians can individualise therapy for patients and provide anticipatory care as situations can alter quite quickly in the last few days of life. Each GP should download their local version to their work desktop. *General Practice Today* is not a textbook of palliative care therapy so the various medications and managements are not further discussed here.

Useful resource for palliative care: Palliative and End of Life Care Guidelines Symptom control for cancer and noncancer patients 2016 North of England Clinical Networks at: http://www.nescn.nhs.uk/wp-content/uploads/2016/09/NECNXPALLIATIVEXCAREX2016.pdf.

DEATH CERTIFICATION

Ultimately, we will all end up mentioned on a death certificate which one of our family members will probably collect from our GP, the hospital or, occasionally, coroner. Families can see the causes of death, register the death and use them in family history searches. With the certificate they can arrange the funeral and reading of the will. In addition, there is a public health function in accurate filling of the form so the cause of death by age can be recorded to create public health statistics and determine health actions. There is no payment for death certification.

The death certificate is filled in by the GP who attended the person in their last illness and who has access to their patient's records. For patients who have died in hospital, the certifier may be one of several doctors on the medical team, although the consultant has ultimate responsibility. If the GP has not seen the patient for 14 days and not seen the body after death, then they should call the coroner. If a death is unexpected or of unnatural or unknown cause (for example suicide, poisoning or following a fall) or death is from an industrial disease (asbestosis seems the most common in my practice), then the doctor should speak to the coroner's officer. The coroner and her/his officers are very helpful if you want to check items with them. It is usual in these circumstances for the coroner to organise a postmortem and the family should be advised.

It is acceptable, occasionally, to sign old age as a cause of death in the over 80s, but there should not be any other discernible cause of death and again, a phone call to the coroner's office would be wise. In 30 years of practice this has happened on only four occasions. If the cause of death is unknown or due to unnatural causes, including industrial disease, the coroner will arrange a postmortem and this should be mentioned to the family. Our patients with asbestosis know they will have a postmortem, so their families understand the process of certification in this instance before death.

The death certificate has instructions on how to fill it in at the front.

The top line (1a) is the cause of death in pathological or disease terms (not symptoms, like syncope).

The second line (1b) is the underlying cause of death

Part 2 below outlines other significant illnesses or injuries which contributed to death, but not directly.

An example might be

1a) community-acquired pneumonia
1b) lung cancer
1c) smoker
2) left-sided weakness from previous stroke

Cremation forms may need completion. The GP who filled in the death certificate will also complete and sign the cremation form 4 in England. This GP then asks an independent GP (not a practice partner) who has been qualified for five years to fill in form 5. The GPs discuss the case and give the form 5 GP access to the patient's notes and investigations so that she/he is also satisfied as to the cause of death. Any implants at all, loop recorders, ICDs, pacemakers, intramedullary orthopaedic nails and implants such as drug pumps, etc. need to be reported before cremation and removed. It is important to fulfil the instructions on the form exactly and examine the body carefully. Doctors do receive a fee for cremation forms. It is important to fill these forms out as soon as possible for the sake of the grieving family.

Useful resources for end of life care:

- Treatment and care towards the end of life: good practice in decision making – GMC 2010 at: http://www.gmc-uk.org/guidance/ethical_guidance/end_of_life_care.asp.
- Carers UK website Managing someone's affairs at: https://www.carersuk.org/help-and-advice/practical-support/managing-someone-s-affairs This is a good site for our carers.
- Making decisions: A guide for advice workers The Mental Capacity Act 2005 at: https://www.gov.uk/government/publications/advice-workers-mental-capacity-act-decisions.
- Care of dying adults in the last days of life NICE guidelines [NG31] Published date: December 2015 at: https://www.nice.org.uk/guidance/ng31.
- 2017/18 General Medical Services (GMS) contract Quality and Outcomes Framework (QOF) Guidance for GMS contract 2016/17 at: http://www.nhsemployers.org/~/media/Employers/Documents/Primary%20care%20contracts/QOF/2017-18/201718%20Quality%20and%20outcomes%20framework%20summary%20of%20changes.pdf.
- The Gold Standards framework at: http://www.goldstandardsframework.org.uk/advance-care-planning.

- Death certification Guidance for doctors completing Medical Certificates of Cause of Death in England and Wales by Office for National Statistics' Death Certification Advisory Group, Revised July 2010 advice at: https://www.gro .gov.uk/Images/medcert_July_2010.pdf.
- Cremation guidance at: https://www.gov.uk/government/uploads/system /uploads/attachment_data/file/325750/cremation-doctors-guidance.pdf.

Confidentiality

If a patient has capacity it is up to them to talk about their medical issues with their family and friends; a doctor cannot divulge a patient's problem to others. What occurs between the doctor and their patient is confidential. If maintaining confidentiality places someone else at risk, so that there is a need to divulge a confidence in order to protect others, then the GP should seek advice. In the greater public interest confidentiality may be breached; but the doctor should tell the patient he/she is going to do this. This is only fair, unless doing so would endanger the GP or another HCP. The GMC has again excellent guidance and case-studies on confidentiality and the e-address is at the end of the confidentiality discussion under 'useful resources'. Most information which we are privileged to hear as doctors will go to our graves with us and confidentiality will be respected.

I am going to highlight a few important issues which have taxed myself and colleagues over the years.

Practice staff need retraining periodically to keep any information they hear or see confidential. This is more difficult for them than for GPs, as they are more likely to live in the practice area and know the patients and local happenings. They are more likely to be asked about happenings by their friends and relatives and it might be easy to let a confidence slip out unintentionally.

Sometimes relatives ask GPs not to discuss a patient's illness, e.g. cancer diagnosis, with the patient, as it leaves the patient 'very upset when you have gone'. However, GPs have a duty to discuss the cancer with the patient unless 'serious harm' might ensue but even then, they should periodically review the decision. It is difficult to pretend a patient hasn't got an aggressive cancer when the patient's health is deteriorating. People are not stupid and deserve thoughtful consultations. In general, being open and honest is the best default position. This also applies to children and young people, if the GP feels they have capacity and want to know more about their illness.

Sometimes it is not the illness doctors are asked to hide but the source of concern. It is very difficult to visit a patient when a relative has asked the GP to visit with concerns 'but don't tell them I spoke to you'. I usually counter that I will not state the requesters identity unless I have to. I am happy to visit a patient and ask how they are, but if it is clear that I can only have obtained information from a family member, e.g. about erratic driving or a recent blackout, then it may be better to come clean and tell the patient. Therefore, let the concerned caller know you cannot guarantee anonymity. I have never had problems with this position.

However, there are big happenings and 'secrets' which are probably impossible to keep confidential. When something traumatic or exceptional happens it is very difficult for anyone not to tell another person about it, regardless of guidance and the law. It would be helpful for health care systems to be realistic and provide space for limited disclosure when absolutely necessary but this is not offered at present. Be aware of this; it is important. Some things will always be so upsetting or surprising that not everyone can 'keep them in'. The GMC make it clear that GPs must maintain confidentiality. The GP or HCP should consider the effects on another of discussing an 'exceptional happening.' Will debriefing to a trusted senior colleague maintain confidentiality or make it more likely to be further breached? In the circumstance of needing to tell someone, due to upset, then I would suggest meeting the senior partner as there may be issues of future patient management that also need discussing. In addition, the patient may be discussed anonymously initially.

It is also important to keep patient's record access cards and codes safe and not share them, even if someone has forgotten theirs and asks for yours as a favour. The GP should log out at end of the clinic so that notes are not accessible to anyone else entering the room.

Requests for reports on patients or sending off their notes should have the patient's signed informed consent documented within a reasonable time-frame. I have seen solicitor claims for road accidents on which the patient's signature is over 12 months old on a few occasions. In this situation ask the solicitor to provide updated signed consent from their client. Do check if patients have signed to see reports or their records before they are sent off or not. If you notice, or perhaps know through consultations, that an unrelated aspect which is personal to the patient, e.g. they have had a difficult time in their marriage, they have been tested for HIV, etc., is in the records then you should check with the patient whether the person asking for a copy of the patient records can receive all the information or whether some is irrelevant and should be excluded.

GP records should not be altered. If a GP decides to add to a patient record after the consultation has finished and the patient has left, then they must make a new entry. Never change records after the event. This has got doctors into trouble and even prison.

Scenario: Tempted to alter records
Mrs X, 41 years old, comes in with indigestion to see a GP and is found dead the next day at home. The family feel the doctor missed an acute myocardial infarction. The GP looks at the notes, feeling very upset for the patient and anxious for him/herself. The GP has never had a complaint before and now feels panicky. The GP remembers that the patient said antacids like Gaviscon had helped the pain but hasn't written it in the record and wants to add it in now to the entry from the day before....

Stop – this just cannot be done.

The GP can write a new entry stating the current date, what has happened to the patient and that he/she wants to add a memo from memory but he/she cannot alter the original entry. If records are altered, what else has the doctor altered? What else about that doctor can be believed? Just never do it.

Scenario: Wanting to let a colleague know (and confidentiality)

Mr Y comes into the GP surgery and pulls a kitchen knife out. After the GP tells him she is scared he apologises and tells the GP that it was just to show how bad he felt and how close he had come to suicide in the last week. He places it on the GP's desk and leaves it there. The GP deals with the situation, helps Mr Y, and is left at the end of the consultation with the knife in her possession on the desk and just needs to tell someone!

This is an ideal situation to talk through with a senior colleague. There are issues of self-harm, subsequent management, and what the GP is going to do with the knife (it won't exactly fit the sharp box)! The GP needs to discuss if the patient is a hazard to anyone else and of course how they are feeling about the episode. Later there would be discussion about future consultations with this patient and safety. Thoughts and actions can be checked with medical defence bodies, who are always willing to talk through difficulties and best actions.

Some patients are prone to violence or outbursts and are managed under a safe haven scheme. In this scenario though the patient was a gentle soul, known over many years to the practice and had genuinely come to show the weapon he had been considering using on himself. He was appalled that the doctor might feel threatened and very apologetic. People should be thought about as individuals.

Scenario: Gossip from hospital reaches GP practice and the patient

Mr Y has complications from routine surgery and receives 30 units of blood. The GP knows because his GP registrar tells him about the case as several hospital staff have been upset by it and have discussed it. Mr Y comes for a sick note and relates that his cousin knew about his post-operative bleeding as his cousin's best friend is a nurse at the hospital. He can't remember being ill himself but isn't happy that he appears to have been a source of gossip. Asked if he wants to make a complaint he says no – he just wanted to off load this to the GP.

In this scenario, the doctor has a duty to let the GP registrar know that the patient is upset about lack of confidentiality and send that message back to colleagues. The GP may take it up with the hospital but only with the patient's consent. The patient doesn't want to make a complaint but it is also reasonable to ensure that practice staff are reminded about confidentiality as they may have heard about this out-of-the-ordinary happening too. That is, practice staff may be privy to local information about patients in the practice through their own networks and require reminding periodically about confidentiality.

There are occasions when a doctor will disclose information in the public interest. These are unusual, and again, always look for senior colleague support and discuss with your defence organisation, who are experienced in these unfamiliar situations.

The most common problem is a patient possibly unfit to drive who continues to do so. The patient may be unfit to drive due to alcoholism, uncontrolled epilepsy, uncontrolled diabetes with a tendency to hypoglycaemia, severe dementia or visual defects, etc. GPs are not the police. It is our job to tell a patient with capacity that they should not drive if that is true. The GP can share the Driver and Vehicle Licensing Authority (DVLA) *Assessing fitness to drive* document on the computer screen with the patient. If the GP tells the patient not to drive they should record the decision in the notes and tell the patient that he/she has done this. This is another excellent desktop resource for doctors: *Assessing fitness to drive: a guide for medical professionals*. Be clear and professional in stating that you have concerns about the patient's fitness to drive, that you are making a note in their records, and that they should inform the DVLA who will then contact them back. Ensure that they know that once the GP has written they are unfit to drive in their records, they are not insured if they get in their car and are driving against medical advice. Most patients will comply and tell you that they will inform the DVLA themselves but some will not. Then, in the public interest, you should tell them that you are going to contact the DVLA on their behalf and again make a note in the patient's records. GPs meet most scenarios over a long career but not often enough to become expert, and so again, a check with your medical defence body is in order. If you are not sure whether a patient is unfit to drive, seek a second opinion.

Scenario: Drunk in clinic
Mr Y is drunk in the clinic and nearly falling off the chair. The GP notices his car keys and asks whether the patient drove there. The patient says, 'Yes'. The GP takes Mr Y's car keys off him to stop him driving home, which he had clearly intended to do. As this patient was a known alcoholic, the GP informed the DVLA and medical defence organisation as the car and keys need some sort of plan!

Here the doctor was in no doubt about the potential harms of inaction.

Scenario: Dementia and dangerous driving
On a domiciliary visit with a psychogeriatrician to a severely demented patient who lived alone and was in denial of his problems, the specialist took his car keys away and arranged emergency disconnection of his gas cooker.

These are rare occurrences but illustrate points about a doctor's responsibility to society. These scenarios and others like them will happen at times.

If a patient with capacity says they will comply with the GP's recommendation, i.e. to inform the DVLA and not to drive (they have a legal obligation to inform them), then confidentiality is respected and a written record made. If the patient lacks capacity or states that they will not comply, or the GP finds that they are still driving, perhaps from a report from a concerned relative, then in the public interest the doctor should inform the authorities.

It can be difficult to comply when the GP feels sympathy for the patient but it is the doctor's duty to obey the law.

Scenario: Hypoglycaemia and driving
Miss X, 28 years old, drives for a living as a successful sales executive and is a type 1 insulin dependent diabetic (T1IDDM). A record from an A&E visit shows that she was admitted with a hypoglycaemic episode. The GP's records

show that this also happened 10 months ago, but did not need admission. The GP asks to see her and shows her the DVLA Assessing fitness to drive: a guide for medical professionals which bars her from driving. This is despite her monitoring her sugars as recommended, because she has had two hypoglycaemic attacks requiring management in 12 months. She is devastated as she has done her best and will lose her job. She asks the GP to 'let her off' and 'turn a blind eye'. The GP has known her all her life and feels terrible but there is a duty of care to society and the GP must follow professional guidance. The patient understands this but is understandably disappointed.

The GMC guidance on confidentiality covers lots of other important scenarios, such as gunshot or knife wounds, but in primary care it can sometimes be difficult to be sure of the risk to society or how to proceed. People tell you strange things sometimes.

Scenario: Gun under the sofa
Mr Y, 23 years old, tells the GP that he has a gun under his sofa. It seemed to just come out in conversation as he was worried about it!

The GP tells the patient that it is the patient's duty to inform the police and take the gun into a police station immediately. The GP phones her defence body for advice and has told Mr Y she is going to do this and that he can phone in to find the result of the advice later. The GP was advised to inform police by her defence body and did so. The patient phoned in later and was informed of this. He told the GP that he was about to hand the gun in later that day anyway and did so.

In some situations, when there is a risk to the GP or staff, patients would not be informed but in this circumstance the GP did not feel at risk.

Scenario: Serious transmissible disease
Mr Y has been diagnosed with HIV and in the original consultation told his GP that he has two sexual partners, one of whom is a partner in the same household and on the practice list.

The GP may assume the infectious diseases team have spoken to him about infectivity, disclosure and safe sex but should check this. If it becomes apparent that the patient is unwilling to protect partners then the GP has a duty of care to the partners of an infectious patient. This is clear in GMC guidance and like all disclosure, the GP would have to let the patient know that he/she intended to break confidentiality in the public interest.

Again, the GP should take advice from the GMC website and their defence body.

These cases relate the principles of confidentiality to general practice difficulties but not exact patient scenarios. They do not expose any patient confidences over the years.

Useful resources:

- GMC Guidance; Confidentiality: good practice in handling patient information (2017) at: http://www.gmc-uk.org/guidance/ethical_guidance /confidentiality.asp
- *Assessing fitness to drive: a guide for medical professionals* from: Driver and Vehicle Licensing Agency (DVLA) at: https://www.gov.uk/guidance /assessing-fitness-to-drive-a-guide-for-medical-professionals

Other commonly encountered rules and regulations

This part of our rules and regulations section highlights some areas which are often not well understood but are commonly met and may contain some pitfalls, so anecdotally have been difficult for young doctors to grasp.

Professionalism is defined by society's expectations of their doctors. To achieve this, we all carry rules and regulations with us like an invisible professional white coat. In order to practice well they are with us but unseen by the patient. Patients do not want doctors motivated by rules, they want knowledgeable doctors who know the rules but who make the care of their patients their first concern; this requires skill and compassion. The front of the coat, the part of you that meets the patient, is therefore plain.

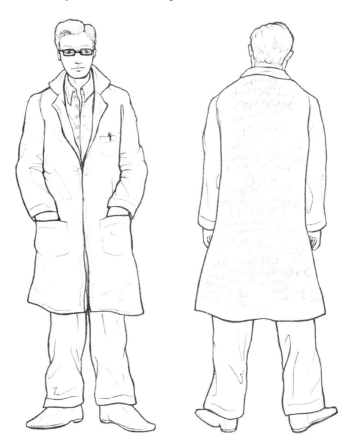

PATIENT GROUP DIRECTIONS (PGDs) AND PATIENT SPECIFIC DIRECTIONS (PSDs)

These are confusing to young doctors and HCPs entering practice in Trusts and primary care. The Human Medicines Regulations 2012 does not allow nurses, or other registered HCPs who are not qualified prescribers, to administer or supply prescription-only-medicines (POMs) unless they have one of the following:

1. Signed prescription.
2. Patient specific direction (PSD). This is a written instruction, signed by the GP, usually for a medicine to be supplied or administered to a named patient after individual assessment by the prescriber.
3. Patient group direction (PGD) is a written instruction signed by the practice lead GP allowing the supply or administration of medicines to groups of patients who may not be individually identified before presentation for treatment.

Scenario for PSD

Mr Smith, 58 years old, attends the GP practice and sees the healthcare assistant (HCA) for his vitamin B12 injection.

This is administered using a PSD.

A PSD is a named prescription. It has the patient's name, drug name, dosage, etc. It is specific to that patient. It does not pertain to a group of patients, conditions or to an unnamed individual. As the prescriber and dispenser are not the same person, it is used so that the GP can delegate the responsibility of the injection to a suitably qualified, trained HCP, provided the GP has assessed the patient as in need of the medication. In the scenario above it is the HCA. This person must have appropriate knowledge, skills and training. The practice must have specific guidelines in place for the HCP to administer by PSD. Other prescribers, like dentists or nurse-prescribers, can delegate administration of medicines by PSD to non-prescribing HCPs. If this scenario was instead that of an HCA in a GP flu clinic, there would have to be a signed list of individual patient names attending in advance, which would need to be checked.

Scenario for PGD

The GP practice runs a flu session, inviting at risk individuals to attend between 12–3 pm on October 17. The non-prescribing nurse administers the influenza jabs using a PGD.

A PGD is a procedure or policy drawn up by a multidisciplinary team which allows the delegation of medicines to an authorised, responsible, appropriately trained and skilled HCP who can then administer to a group of patients without having their names in advance. This group will have a specific clinical condition. In the above scenario, it is patients with conditions causing an increased risk of influenza. HCAs cannot administer medications via PGDs as they are not on the list of professionally regulated authorised persons. Nurses in general practice who are nurse prescribers do not have to work to PSDs or PGDs but non-prescribing nurses require PGDs.

PGDs are sent to practices from Public Health England (in England) and a lead GP signs to authorise which nurses can use the PGD.

PGDs can also be excellent sources of information about indications and contraindications of medications, e.g. immunisations or contraceptives. Medical students, young doctors and young GPs would find them helpful resources so I urge you to ask for copies from your practice manage or clinical commissioning group (CCG). As an aside, PGDs cannot be used in travel clinics for private travel vaccinations and antimalarial tablets. In this instance, the patient requires a PSD if an authorised, trained non-prescriber is running the clinic.

PSDs and PGDs can improve HCPs working interest and skills and save GPs' time. However, any skills that the GP delegates may result in deskilling of that GP and it is up to the GP to decide on which skills they are happy to lose. There is always a down side to every advance!

Useful resources:

- Patient Group Directions MPG 2 Published Aug 2013 at https://www.nice .org.uk/guidance/mpg2
- Nigel's surgery 19: Patient Group Directions (PGDs)/Patient Specific Directions (PSDs) from the CQC website at: https://www.cqc.org.uk/content /nigels-surgery-19-patient-group-directions-pgds-patient -specific-directions-psds

CHAPERONES

An intimate examination such as vaginal, breast, groin or scrotum examinations demand a chaperone but, for some patients, chest and abdominal examinations might be considered intimate as well. Some patients may not be touched by another person from year to year and so a doctor's hand on their body may have more significance than the GP appreciates. Chaperoning also relates to trust. A young doctor, a doctor of the opposite sex, or a doctor unknown to the patient may be seen as a sexual or intrusive doctor and a chaperone helps to keep the doctor safe.

Some patients are surprised when asked whether they want a chaperone; the idea of two people present during the examination rather than one may result in a refusal but always record it in the notes. I have not experienced a difference in chaperone acceptance between men and women patients. Patients should understand that GPs have no personal interest in their bodies when they are being examined; we act as doctors. Debunking ideas of embarrassment for men and women is an effective way of creating professional boundaries. Occasionally a patient might behave in an overtly sexual manner. If a patient tells a dirty joke, then tell the patient that you are sorry but that joke is inappropriate within a doctor-patient relationship and that they need to see a different doctor in the practice if the behaviour continues. Practices often allocate patients to same sex doctors if their behaviour has caused low-level concern.

Scenario: Chaperone refused

Mr Y is 50 years old and comes into the practice, surprised at the GP . The following conversation takes place:

Mr Y: 'Oh, I thought it was a male doctor!'
GP: 'I can phone him to see when he has a gap if you wish?'
Mr Y: 'No, I've got a lump in my scrotum and I'm here now'.
GP after a few questions: 'I am going to wash my hands, put some gloves on and have a look if that is okay? It is easier for me if you are stood up and can lower your pants behind the curtain there. Do you want me to call a chaperone in?'
Mr Y: 'No, thanks. It's just a bit embarrassing'.
GP: 'Not to me – it's a bit of tissue for me to examine. But we have chaperones if you would like one'.
Mr Y who has gone behind curtain: 'No, I'm ready'.
The GP arranged a USS to check, but the lump felt and was a spermatocele.

However, a male GP partner relates that he always calls in a chaperone as he feels more at risk as a man. He relates a visit:

On call one evening Dr Y leant over to examine a child with fever who was laid down on the sofa and overheard the young mum and her girlfriend mention he had a nice bottom. He was surprised to be thought of in a sexual way.

Chaperones should ideally be other HCPs but as they are usually busy seeing patients they can also be general practice trained reception staff. The chaperone should be disclosure and barring service (DBS) checked and have undergone training in patient's rights, in whistle-blowing any concerns, and in understanding their roles and responsibilities. As staff usually live in the practice area, check with patients if they want the particular individual to be the chaperone as they may be friends, relatives, etc. Clear communication is always welcomed by patients and the practice chaperoning policy should be readily accessible.

Recording in the notes keeps the doctors safe.

Just as an extra on chaperoning (as it brings gender to mind), GPs should avoid dressing in a provocative manner. It is obviously inappropriate to send sexual signals out to patients. I have seen female doctors in training videos wearing skirts that revealed their thighs and underwear. It put me off listening and clearly on the video distracted the patient too! The same applies for male GPs who should wear appropriately formal, covered-up clothing. I ask the reader to reflect on dress codes and choose attire that is neutral.

USE OF SOCIAL MEDIA AND PHONES

This is an area all young doctors and opinion leaders need to come to grips with. Online discussion, even on privacy-setting on Facebook pages, constitutes public comment. Facebook is littered with health care worker comments. How anonymous are they?

- *Busy day, I've seen the most disgusting foot.*
- *Exhausted, thought I had finished and then a 2-year-old with just a runny nose comes in – what a waste of time!*
- *I can't stand my practice.............. he's always telling me what to do. Going to open the Prosseco and get pissed.*
- *Such a great night last night, I've been really hung over at work today.*

Any relative of a patient who attended that GP that day with a 'disgusting foot' will recognise who this refers to. It is very hard to completely anonymise activity. Some comments are even more explicit and my advice is that they need to stop.

Many social media comments are put on really to express the doctor's ego state; often to encourage ego building, not to help the patient. These are inappropriate in medicine. Patients, relatives and fellow workers can interpret comments on social media as libel or breaches of professional standards. Before you type, ask yourself, 'is this appropriate?' How would the patient or relative feel if reading this? Separate out your personal and your professional personas.

Derogatory messages on social media about patients or staff are unforgiveable; just don't do it.

Sometimes doctors are approached to be Friends on Facebook with patients, or have had suggestive sexual comments or other personal comments made about them. The author is responsible for their entries and GPs can complain and take action about these. Do not 'Friend' patients on social media as it transcends the doctor-patient relationship.

GPs cannot have a sexual relationship with a patient, even when he/she has left your list, as they may have befriended the GP at a time of vulnerability and accuse him/her of unprofessional behaviour later on. If a GP has genuinely fallen in love, this is more difficult. The couple might wonder how long is 'a long time' after the patient has left the GP list in order to take up a relationship? This is open to interpretation so I recommend referring to GMC guidance if you find yourself becoming seriously attached to a patient and contact your defence body for advice. Emotions occur, the patient needs to become an ex-patient and the emotional difficulties about how you feel need to be discussed with an experienced authority. You will be strongly advised not to embark on a relationship.

Lastly, some short advice about phones. Doctors should assume they are being recorded in surgery. A patient in my practice has phoned up for lab test results pretending to be a GP and played the recording back to me in clinic. One obsessive patient reached into his shirt pocket to turn the recording off as he left. Just assume your conversation is recorded and will be replayed by the patient, perhaps to relatives and friends.

Turn your own phone off or on silent. I have seen doctors responding to a vibration of their phone whilst being videoed for training purposes. The reaction is visible and breaks the concentration of the patient and doctor. Everyone deserves their GP to attend to them fully in their appointment.

A patient once related that when a locum GP's phone went off the GP said, 'Excuse me I just want to make a dinner booking' and did!

Dear me!

COMPLAINTS

Each practice has a complaints procedure which is easily accessible to patients and should be highlighted to them if there is any complaint in the practice. Doctors should be aware and informed about the practice's complaints procedure and the rules for removing patients.

The principles of good complaint handling are simple. Deal with complaints swiftly, take them seriously, be transparent in dealings and be honest. Most people will see their GP at some time, often at a time of stress about their health, and most NHS interactions are in primary care. Therefore, cultures of dealing with complaints when things are perceived to or have actually gone wrong are important. Changing cultures so that we all learn from mistakes and support each other to do better should be the default GP position. Many complaints are solved just by listening. I have twice made formal complaints to our local hospital on behalf, and consented by, patients when standards have been low. At this time, I have wanted to be listened to and have wanted to know that the problem would not be repeated.

Scenario: Patient complaint
Miss X develops a neuralgic problem which doesn't respond to usual GP therapy and is referred to a specialist. The specialist tells her that a new treatment should have been given. The patient writes to the GP complaining that her care was inferior. The GP checks latest guidelines and the specialist's recommendation is not in them. The specialist is contacted and told that a complaint has been made and is asked to justify the comment to the patient. The next OPC letter retracted the suggestion with an acknowledgement that it had caused patient confusion and that the practice management was correct. The practice wrote to the patient explaining that it had looked at the latest evidence but that the management was usual practice. The patient replied saying she was really pleased with the response, was sorry she had complained, but felt the response was great and wanted to put the incident behind her. The issue was discussed at a practice meeting and written up as a significant event.

Had the practice management been outdated though, the practice would have acknowledged this and apologised. Most people just want an apology.

Scenario: Patient complaint

A patient pursued an OOH organisation complaining about poor care. In effect, she had been coerced into attending OOH by taxi and then did not receive care. There had been no adverse health sequelae. She continued with her complaint and eventually the OOH's manager met with her and asked, 'What would you like me to do?'

The patient's response was, 'I would like an apology and I would like the £20 taxi money refunding'.

The complaint had cost a lot more in staff typing and reading time than £20. In this circumstance, the patient's complaint about a wasted journey was accurate, none of us were disputing this. We understood the patient's point of view and the OOH manager reimbursed the £20 and the patient was satisfied.

Scenario: Patient complaint

Mr Y attended to say he felt his partner's terminal cancer had been badly handled over a few weeks before diagnosis.

The patient had attended the practice repeatedly but had not been given a follow up appointment with the same, or indeed any doctor. Despite a complaint of weight loss, she had not been weighed.

The problem had been different doctors and a lack of continuity. The patient was reluctant to reattend and this had created a lot of tension at home. I can only imagine the angst this man felt in persuading his partner to reattend, as she was frightened of the diagnosis she might be given. The GP asked what the complainant wanted to happen and outlined options, including a formal complaint against the practice. In this case Mr Y and the GP acknowledged that he might go to a legal professional for litigation. The GP said he would speak to the practice doctors to ensure it didn't happen again anyway. Mr Y decided he wanted the GP to pursue the last option only. He wanted to know that the doctors all knew they had let him and his partner down and that they would learn from it. The practice did and sent the complainant a letter outlining what had been done to improve with an apology. Subsequently he has felt able to use the practice services again.

GPs meet all sorts of people and whilst no one is 'normal' and most people are absolutely wonderful, there are also some personalities which are very difficult to manage and take up an inordinate amount of the practice time with complaints. Some people set out to complain. Some people are supercilious, antagonistic or just plain rude to their doctors and staff. Some people cannot control their anger. Some people take up legal claims continually. All these stress the local society in which they live, including the GP practice. It might help the reader to acknowledge that being reported to the GMC for no true reason is awful but maybe the patient is also suing their neighbour for renewing their garden fence, the council for tripping up on a kerbstone, and has an exaggerated road traffic accident personal injury claim ongoing too. Some people cause havoc and this is not yet well-recognised and acknowledged by the organisations governing GPs. Unfortunately, such people don't come with a clear warning label and cause many GPs to go off with stress, retire and very occasionally even take their own lives. My advice with difficult patients is that they should be discussed at practice meetings with a small group of colleagues (meetings come in all sizes); the practice staff must be protected and supported against poor behaviour and know that it is very important to follow complaints procedures correctly because these people are experts and will complain if you don't comply with processes.

There are counselling services for doctors and all doctors should be registered with an independent GP; not a spouse, not a practice partner. A practice coming together to manage a difficult problem is the best support. Often issues have run out of control before the problem is recognised. As with much general practice, early recognition and discussion of potential problems would improve case management and support colleagues in difficult situations.

Doctors receive updates and circulars from their defence bodies. It seems to take postgraduate doctors about 15 years (anecdotally!) before they read through these sensibly and learn from them. I have known GP trainees to admit that these go in recycling unopened. Yet these circulars act as an early warning system and highlight rare conditions, presentations and pitfalls in practice. I strongly recommend a culture shift from fear to learning, talking problems through and, if things go wrong, not avoiding but supporting colleagues. There should be a culture of supporting each other in practice even when this may dent the rest of the team's confidence.

In addition, when practice care has gone well then this should also be disseminated and discussed. Doctors should not beat themselves up about lack of perfection, but enjoy doing a good job.

Useful resources:

- An opportunity to improve General practice complaint handling across England: a thematic review 03/16 at https://www.ombudsman.org.uk/news-and-blog/news/new-report-puts-gp-complaint-handling-spotlight-and-shows-practices-how-do-it
- The related site has a briefer top 10 tips at: https://www.ombudsman.org.uk/sites/default/files/Tips_for_general_practice_leaflet_1.pdf.

ABORTION AND THE LAW

The 1967 Abortion Act amended by the Human Fertilisation and Embryology Act (HFEA) 1990 applies to England, Scotland and Wales. Over 90% of abortions are provided by the NHS, often by independent sector organisations working under NHS contracts. Half of teenage pregnancies end in abortion, also called terminations of pregnancy (ToP), but have reduced to the lowest level since records began in England and Wales. Therefore, be aware that not everyone attending with a positive pregnancy test has a wanted pregnancy.

Women have a choice of

- Continuing with the pregnancy and bringing the child up
- Continuing and having the child adopted or fostered
- Having an abortion

Some women access their abortion (bypassing the GP), by going directly to abortion service providers who provide the signatures for the abortion act. Some women who would like an abortion may unfortunately ask a GP who has a conscientious objection to abortion and so does not feel able to give unbiased care. If this occurs then the GP must provide the woman with an alternative doctor, without delay, who will assess the request in a neutral and professional manner. In addition, this information should be in the practice leaflet or online practice site.

Consent to abortion is straightforward provided the individual has capacity. Children under 13 years old who request an abortion are judged to have been raped and require reporting and safeguarding intervention. Children aged 13–16 years old can consent to abortion if, in the GP's view, they conform to the Fraser guidelines. The GP should encourage them to talk about the pregnancy with their parents or a trusted adult but if they have capacity to consent and do not want to, they are entitled to the procedure and to confidentiality. Young people 16–17 years old, who have capacity, can consent and have rights of confidentiality (although it is good practice to involve parents for support if the young woman agrees to this. If they do not then again, confidentiality should be respected). The GP should ensure that the pregnancy is unwanted and that the girl has a nonabusive relationship.

Abortion is illegal after 24 weeks of gestation. Abortion law is clear (usually) when a fetus has been found to have a severe defect. However, difficulties have arisen with the definition of severe deformity. In practice though, most abortions are due to adverse social or mental issues and signed on the logic that to continue a pregnancy is always more risky than early termination of a pregnancy and that the woman states that an unwanted child would affect her mental health adversely. Section C, below, accounts for 97% of abortion act form completions.

Statutory grounds for ToP section C:

C. The pregnancy has not exceeded its 24th week and the continuance of the pregnancy would involve risk, greater than if the pregnancy were terminated, of injury to the physical or mental health of the pregnant woman: Section 1(1)(a). *

Women are offered a choice of methods for ToP depending on the technical aspects of gestation and any unusual maternal factors. ToP may be medical, using mifepristone and then misoprostol, or surgical, using vacuum aspiration, or, in later gestations, dilation and evacuation. The guidelines from the Royal College of Obstetricians and Gynaecologists (RCOG) recommend consent, counselling, discussion of failure and complication rates, all of which are very unusual. Blood

---

* Abortion Act 1967 at: http://www.legislation.gov.uk/ukpga/1967/87/section/1

for Group and Rhesus status is taken and antiD administered at the end of the procedure if she is Rhesus negative. The woman should also be asked about her risks of STI, and symptoms and swabs for chlamydia taken. Prophylactic antibiotics for chlamydia and anaerobes, e.g. azithromycin and metronidazole, are given. There is also a discussion of ongoing contraception, perhaps an intrauterine device (IUCD) inserted at the time of ToP, so there is a lot for a patient to take in. For the clinician in the ToP clinic there are a number of factors to be thought through and discussed with the patient in order to offer best care.

Useful resources:

- The Law and Ethics of Abortion BMA Views November 2014 at https://www.bma.org.uk/advice/employment/ethics/ethics-a-to-z/abortion
- The Care of Women Requesting Induced Abortion Evidence-based Clinical Guideline Number 7 RCOG Nov 2011 at: https://www.rcog.org.uk/globalassets/documents/guidelines/abortion-guideline_web_1.pdf.

FEMALE GENITAL MUTILATION (FGM)

The Female Genital Mutilation Act 2003 in England, Wales and Northern Ireland and the Prohibition of Female Genital Mutilation (Scotland) Act 2005 in Scotland state that FGM is illegal. It was amended in 2015 by the Serious Crimes Act to introduce mandatory reporting of FGM in girls below 18 years of age by HCPs, including GPs, and others to social workers and the police. This has made GPs more aware of their responsibilities. FGM refers to any procedure involving partial or total removal of the external female genitalia (often clitoris) and so varies in amount of resulting disfigurement, functional and sexual problems. There are no health benefits for girls with FGM. It can be a common practice in some African, Far and Middle Eastern countries and so may be continued when people arrive in the UK as accepted practice. Health Education England has an excellent e-learning for health (e-LfH) module on this topic which I recommend. It can affect 1.5% of antenatal women but rates vary and in 2004 were reported as high as 6% in inner London and 2% in Manchester.* Some FGM will be so severe that the baby needs to be born by Caesarean section as the incredible elasticity of the external genitalia is lost. It is one of the wonders of nature that a vaginal entrance can expand at birth to allow a 9–10 cm fetal skull width through, often without any tearing of the tissues. A woman who has had FGM and is over 18 years old may require assessment of sequelae, e.g. psychological effects, difficulties with conception, pregnancy or urinary infections. A woman over 18 years old does not

* A Statistical Study to Estimate the Prevalence of Female Genital Mutilation in England and Wales. Summary Report Foundation for Women's Health, Research and Development (FORWARD) In collaboration with The London School of Hygiene and Tropical Medicine and The Department of Midwifery, City University Funded by Department of Health, England Principal Investigators Efua Dorkenoo, Linda Morison, Alison Macfarlane. At: http://forwarduk.org.uk/wp-content/uploads/2016/01/PREVALENCE-STUDY_FORWARD_25_01_08.pdf.

need to be reported to social services and on to the police but anyone under 18 does need reporting. The GP may talk to an adult woman and discover that there are younger girls at risk of undergoing FGM, in the UK or being sent abroad for the procedure, perhaps younger sisters or cousins within the family. FGM in the UK or abroad is illegal and GPs must report this possibility to social services as part of their child safe-guarding role. This requires sensitive but firm handling as an act of FGM might have occurred to the patient years prior and be considered by the victim as a part of growing up within her society but is then relabelled as illegal and abusive in our society. The woman may however have always considered it an abuse. I am not condoning FGM but some sensitivity to women from different backgrounds, exploring their feelings and attitudes to FGM, is required within the consultation. Many women feel they have been abused but some may never have considered FGM as abuse and may have difficulty accepting FGM as an illegal act.

DISCUSSION ON SAFE-GUARDING, COERCIVE BEHAVIOUR, AND 'MANDATORY' TRAINING

GPs train in child safe-guarding, adult safe-guarding, and domestic violence. These items are also available as e-learning, e.g. e-LfH modules and clinical governance CCG experts also provide locality training. Each practice has a named safe-guarding lead who has expertise and is very helpful in discussing concerns. Child abuse may be sexual, psychological, physical or by neglect. I am not going into the details of these here and have no objection to updates but want to highlight problems with expected updates which have mushroomed over the last decade. Updates can take hours of GP time at little improvement in care as the items, though important, are not common for each GP. Finding the amount of time to update and choosing updates which are useful and relevant is tricky. It is equally important to diagnose a heart attack, an abused child or a suicidal teenager. Anyone can approach primary care with the view that GPs should be experts in all topics but this is impossible. To counter perceived knowledge and skill gaps lots of 'mandatory' training has popped up. As the topics all have high moral value, GPs feel powerless to refuse them. However, many GPs do not see abused children despite years of practice. To have awareness of abuse is very helpful but if an abused child does not come through the clinic door reasonably frequently then the GP will not be particularly skilled despite updates. Phone numbers, emails and forms to fill out will not be immediately memorable or accessible and may have been updated.

In essence, when considering safe-guarding, the questions to consider are as follows:

- Are there safe-guarding issues for this person?
- Are there safe-guarding issues for other members of society, especially children or in pregnancy?
- Is there an immediate danger?
- Is this a criminal, i.e. illegal act?

- Am I contacting the police, social services, getting advice from other agencies, e.g. defence body, partners, safe-guarding lead?
- Have I disclosed my actions to the patient and if not, can I justify this?

Mandatory training is part of a bigger conversation about how to keep up-to-date. Mandatory training currently appears to cover hand washing, infection control, fire safety, governance training, information technology handling, etc. and is presently out of hand. It consumes hours of time, including clinical time, but it is also difficult to suggest an alternative solution without a major overhaul of general practice. It is a consequence of control, made easy by computerisation so that 'doers' are easily audited, managed and at risk of censure if noncompliant. This whole training economy needs a careful overhaul by collaboration of the various regulatory bodies such as RCGP, GMC, Care Quality Commission, NICE, QoF, appraisal and revalidation processes, CCGs, Local Education Training Boards with their deaneries, etc.

Laws do change and there have been great improvements in well-being as a result. Over the last generation physical punishment has become an offence; it is not allowed to smack children or cane them at school. It was usual for patients as young people, but who are now over 50 years old, to see annoyed mums smacking their children in public. A patient of 60 years old related that he was caned for laughing in the school playground at 11 years old! A number of adults in GP clinics reflect that their own upbringing would bring in social service investigation by today's society standards and older doctors need to be aware of the changes and move with and support societal norms.

The Serious Crime Act 2015 creates a new offence of controlling or coercive behaviour in intimate or familial relationships. This might be repeated psychological bullying, including by Internet, physical intimidation, preventing freedom of movement to partners and other family members so that they suffer physical or psychological harm.

The cross-government definition of domestic violence and abuse outlines controlling or coercive behaviour as follows:

- *Controlling behaviour is: a range of acts designed to make a person subordinate and/or dependent by isolating them from sources of support, exploiting their resources and capacities for personal gain, depriving them of the means needed for independence, resistance, and escape and regulating their everyday behaviour.*
- *Coercive behaviour is: a continuing act or a pattern of acts of assault, threats, humiliation, and intimidation or other abuse that is used to harm, punish or frighten their victim.**

* Controlling or Coercive Behaviour in an Intimate or Family Relationship Statutory Guidance Framework December 2015. Home Office at: https://www.gov.uk/government/uploads/system/uploads/attachment_data/file/482528/Controlling_or_coercive_behaviour_-_statutory_guidance.pdf.

Scenario: Abusive behaviour
Miss X, 35 years old, comes for a cervical screening test and tells the practice nurse that she has been kept prisoner in an upstairs flat by her partner for six months and is not allowed out without him. He has not assaulted her but she states that she wants her freedom back, has no money and is frightened of him. He locks her in when he leaves the flat. The partner is in the waiting room of the practice.

This is abusive coercive behaviour.

The patient should be moved to another room in case the partner comes looking for her and the police should be called.

Scenario: Parental bullying
Miss X is is 10 years old and is brought to the GP by mum with a four-month history of bed-wetting. The girl looks sad. There are no other symptoms and there appears to be no problems at home or school. The mum and girl agree to mum leaving the room whilst a few personal questions are asked. When asked whether anyone is ever mean to her or upsets her she relates that her dad has changed her name to "Useless" and never uses her real name. She is frightened of him and never does anything right as far as he is concerned.

This constitutes psychological abuse and coercive behaviour.

Internet bullying, displaying personal (often naked) photos without permission, and stalking, including online, are also offences but it is of course impossible for GPs to be legal experts. However, I mention them so that the reader asks the question *'Is this illegal?'*, and if not sure, asks an authority. Often this is our defence body but might be an expert in the practice, social services or the police, depending upon the circumstances.

The Mental Health Act (MHA) 1983 (Review 2007)

A rather daunting thought as a GP registrar, or newly qualified GP, is sectioning a patient. For those GPs who have not worked in psychiatry, the first time we attend a mental health assessment for proposed section can be nerve-wracking. Are we making the right decision for the patient, their family, their carers and the wider community? We are supported by the MHA, which in turn supports patients to recover mental health when very ill or in crisis, and protects their right to freedom when reasonable. The MHA refers to the legal framework in England and Wales which defines when a patient with a mental disorder can be admitted, detained and treated for a mental health disorder without their consent. If a patient agrees to admission they are a voluntary patient but if sectioned, they are termed 'formal' or 'involuntary' patients. Sectioning is implemented when a patient's mental health puts their own or another person's safety under threat and that person refuses admission or treatment. We use the term 'section' as the different 'sections' of the MHA detail the circumstances and personnel required in order to lawfully detain the patient. Scotland and Northern Ireland have their own laws about compulsory treatment for mental ill health.

MHA DISCUSSION AND SECTIONING

Most GPs will use section 2 (see table below) and those working in OOH settings or in remote locations may use section 4. GPs may be asked to assess patients they know on psychiatric wards to agree to a section 3. Patients may come home on a Community Treatment Order (CTO) to ensure they have follow-up and therapy. Before summarising the sections in a table below we describe the initially confusing array of individuals who may be involved.

1. A GP without any specialised mental health training. Some GPs train to be section 12 approved (see 3).
2. An approved mental health professional (AMHP) is a social worker, mental health nurse, occupational therapist or psychologist who has received special training to help decide whether people need to be admitted to hospital. They are approved by a local social services authority for five years and then need to renew training. Usually they are social workers.
3. A doctor who is approved under Section 12 of the MHA is approved as having special expertise in the diagnosis and treatment of mental health. Section 12 approved doctors (as below) are required for sections 2 and 3 of the MHA.
4. An approved clinician is a doctor, psychologist, mental health nurse, occupational therapist or social worker who has been trained and approved to have responsibility for a patient who has been sectioned in hospital or is on a CTO. They are their main 'responsible clinician'. This approval is renewed by training every five years.

Usually it is possible to admit a patient to hospital with a severe mental health illness without a section, but occasionally it is necessary. The pros and cons of detention and treatment, listening and taking the patient's views into account should be followed if possible. In this way, a case which a GP thought required a section can sometimes convert to a voluntary admission.

Scenario: Patient wants admission – no section needed

Mr Y is 25 years old and sees you with his friend. The friend is concerned about how anxious he is. He hasn't slept for days and is exhausted. He isn't eating and lives alone. This behaviour occurred about eight weeks ago and his friend has been round regularly to help him. When the GP asks Mr Y whether he has unusual thoughts or happenings he finds that Mr Y is sure that there will be a terrorist attack in his town because the TV is sending him messages about this. There is a parked car outside his house, which is watching him. He is afraid to go out. He is hearing voices telling him that as soon as he goes out of the flat the terrorist attack will happen so he has shut himself in to protect everybody. The GP notes that he looks tired, thin and appears to be responding to something or someone invisible behind him. His friend confirms his recent weight loss. When asked whether he would like to be in a hospital as a safe place to have some specialised care he is pleased and says he feels he needs help. An ambulance is called to ensure he arrives safely and he and his friend are given a cup of tea by a staff member who discretely has been asked to check that they remain in the health centre. He agrees to return to the GP when out of hospital to check he is feeling better.

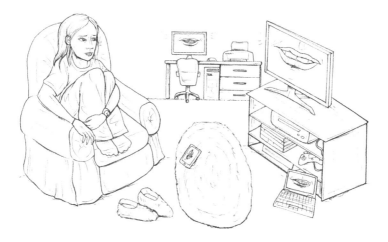

The table below summarises the MHA sections, giving a brief outline of other types of sections that are used for inpatients or by the police:

Section	Who can apply	Who can assess	Duration
Intention: Admit for assessment			
2	AMHP or relative	2 doctors (at least 1 is section 12 approved)	28 days
Intention: Detain for treatment			
3	AMHP	2 doctors (at least 1 is section 12 approved)	6 months
Intention: Admit for urgent assessment from community setting			
4	AMHP or relative	1 doctor	75 hours
Intention: To enter private dwelling to remove patient to place of safety			
135	Police	Police	72 hours
Intention: Remove from public place to a place of safety (usually police station or A&E)			
136	Police	Police	72 hours
Urgent detention of inpatient			
5(2)		1 Doctor	72 hours
Intention: Urgent detention of mental health inpatient			
5(4)		Registered Mental Health Nurse	6 hours

Section 2 is the most commonly used section. This is invoked by an AMHP or a close relative of the patient, and requires an assessment and agreement by two doctors, at least one of which must be section 12 approved, the other can be the patient's GP. There is a form that requires completion and a fee can be claimed. This section is for a maximum of 28 days and is for assessment. This can be extended whilst the patient is an inpatient following assessment and completion of a section 3.

A section 4 is performed in an emergency setting when the GP or section 12 approved doctor cannot wait for a second doctor to assess the patient, due to patient or bystander safety being at risk. This can be invoked by an AMHP or a patient's relative and allows detention of a patient for up to 72 hours for assessment. After assessment by a second doctor (section 12 approved), this can be converted to a section 2 if deemed necessary. The assessment can take place anywhere – usually the patient's home if it is considered safe – but it could be in a clinic or even a hospital. The GP could be asked to attend A&E or even a ward to section a patient, as their GP. If the environment is not safe, then the police may be involved, usually called by the AMHP who has applied for the section.

The assessment itself is usually in the form of a consultation, an interview with the two doctors and AMHP present, along with the patient and any carers or relatives that they wish to have present. A psychiatric history is taken and particular attention is paid to recent events that have led to the section application. After the decision to section is made, the history and reason for the section is documented on the form. If both doctors agree, they then sign and date the form and transport for the patient is arranged to take him/her to the nearest mental health ward that has bed availability.

Like adults, a young person aged under 18 years old, who is mentally ill, has the right to say what they think should happen when adults are making decisions about them. Their opinions should be considered. They have the right to be informed and to be given information, so long as it doesn't cause harm to them. These principles accord with good practice throughout this laws and regulations section. Once sectioned, patients can appeal the section so, as always, excellent record keeping is required. If called to a ward to section a patient who a specialist has deemed as requiring further section, you do not have to complete the section if you do not think it is reasonable. In this circumstance, phone the consultant to ensure you have all the facts. I have occasionally been asked to assess inpatients (IP) who were willing to remain IPs on a voluntary basis, so the ending of one section is not grounds to start a new one.

Scenario: Using emergency section 2

Mr Y is 61 years old and his wife asks the GP to see him over his depression. There is no relevant PMH and the wife cannot persuade him to attend the GP's clinic. On arrival, the patient is building an altar with scissors and knives and praying on the floor in the kitchen. The GP takes a history from the wife in another room and it appears that he has been in a low mood for a couple of weeks but then started to act oddly. He is not eating, roams about at night talking to himself and thinks she is trying to poison him. The GP would have attended with the police if aware of the knives and as the patient is agitated the GP beats a hasty retreat, calls the mental health team and an AMHP and second doctor attends with the GP and with the police. The patient is assessed and sectioned using a section 2 for a 28-day assessment. The patient became agitated at the idea of leaving the house and the police needed to escort him safely to hospital. He was diagnosed with new-onset schizophrenia and had a good response to treatment.

Scenario: GP attends hospital to section patient

Mrs X is 80 years old and lives with her sister. She is losing weight, anorexic, and has no energy. She appears very depressed with flat affect and motor slowing. The GP performed blood tests which came back as normal. She and her sister deny that she is depressed. Review is arranged. Four weeks after the initial onset of depression her sister asks the GP to visit as she won't get out of bed. She is clearly very depressed and a section 2 is arranged after asking the mental health team to visit, as neither the sister or the patient thinks she requires hospital admission. The psychiatrist subsequently asks the GP to visit her as an IP to convert the section 2 to a section 3 as she requires further treatment, possibly electroconvulsive therapy (ECT), as she has not responded to medication. When the GP interviews her the patient is in bed with her face to the wall. She says she wants to go home and does not need any treatment. Within the conversation, she says she does not believe she is a woman but is a dog and needs to go for a long walk. The GP agrees with the section 3 but she does not make much of a response to any therapy and remains in a mental health ward. Sadly, her sister makes an appointment especially to apologise that she hadn't agreed with the GP that her sister was depressed.

Useful resource:

- MIND pages on Mental Health Act and sectioning at: http://www.mind.org .uk/information-support/legal-rights/sectioning/about-sectioning/#three

By the end of this first section on laws and regulations we should have an overview of the external rules which we bring with us into a consultation.

Now let's look at consultations themselves.

2

The consultation

It is more than words...

Practices manage consultations in many different ways and there has never been more choice for patients in accessing primary health care, e.g. online systems, telephone calls, or face-to-face in clinics or on home visits. This consultation section explores the processes of consulting and how these may affect the patient accessing the GP. In addition, this section highlights specific skills that GPs might employ to manage the various consultations and also explores some of the tensions around workload and occasional difficult consultations.

This section introduces the Inner Consultation but does not review all consultation models.

What is a consultation?

The consultation is a private interaction between patients and their health care providers (HCPs). It is the lynch pin of medicine and undoubtedly the most interesting aspect for general practitioners (GPs), who act primarily as medical detectives, analysing information and connecting with the person in front of them to consider possible diagnoses for the plethora of symptoms and signs with which that patient has presented. Think of this section as a modus operandi. For a discussion of confidentiality and consent, please see the laws and regulations section. The consultation is the core of general practice and if we devolve this function to take up other roles, e.g. university posts, primary care medical educators (PCMEs), postgraduate directors, clinical commissioning groups (CCGs), clinical senates, inspection bodies, legal work, etc. we also devolve our medicine to a plethora of other HCPs who already carry out excellent consultations in practices up and down the UK. Taking up a portfolio career and dropping off consultations can be very rewarding and enhance clinical practice but the sequelae must be thought through at a personal and at a national level.

The consultation is currently under threat from pressures to reduce NHS costs and a growing concept of the consultation as somehow inferior to other tasks and so capable of deconstruction into parts that can be delegated to other HCPs and to artificial intelligence (AI) systems. Patients tell us repeatedly that they are more than the sum of their deconstructed patient journeys. Throughout this book we weave the external issues, which improve our practice, into this core section. Everything else – guidelines, laws, regulations, government policy changes – is secondary to the problems which people are presenting to their doctors in an untriaged manner. This is different to hospital-based care (aside from A&E clinicians). In general practice it is unusual for people to arrive with a diagnosis; making accurate diagnoses is our core GP skill. Those of us who see patients, those of us who have been ill, those of us who have watched illness, know that the consultation is key. It is remembered and repeated, and can enhance or distress our lives as patients and clinicians. All doctors love the science of medicine but for most learners and GPs, meeting patients is an equal pleasure. If you like science but you don't like people, then general practice is not going to suit you and you should find another path. Conversely, if you are a great consulter and love people but have little clinical knowledge, general practice is not going to suit you either!

We and our patients hope for a cure or improvement so that patients can function optimally. A second type of GP consultation and professional thinking departs from making primary diagnoses, moving away from the detective role, to supporting people with illnesses for the long term. This requires different consultation skills and processes, though the detective aspect remains accessible if needed.

GPs are trained in several different consultation models. These explore patient data collection through history taking, examination, and investigations to reach a diagnosis. These models direct and explore our discussions with the patient, helping us create management plans and discuss expected outcomes. This book explores the examination and investigation aspects of the consultation as well as history taking. Various factors occur around consultations relating to time and processes for GPs and patients, and many factors within consultations relate to patients' and GPs' beliefs and behaviours. Below I discuss different types of consultations related by doctors and patients over decades before discussing the consultation skills which usually provide satisfactory consultation outcomes for doctors and patients. That is, consultations are different things at different times and to different people.

As GPs we can learn from good practice but also from error. Looking at 'less-than-best practice' is a great way to avoid pitfalls and self-improve. As such, I have included common consultation pitfalls along the way. That said, I want to make it clear that excellent consultations and general practice occur up and down the country for thousands of people every day. I am not complaining about normal high standard general practices and practitioners! The discussion below is not a potted guide to being a GP, nor is it a complete guide to history taking. It is an illustration of types of histories and associated skills which we maintain and improve over our careers.

When people become patients, they give up different degrees of autonomy to gain an explanation and therapy for their symptoms or signs. This is the most important step for lots of people and they have often discussed their symptoms and worries with their friends or relatives ahead of the consultation, and increasingly looked online. There are a few patients who attend too readily, coming with trivia, e.g. *'What do you think about this cracked finger nail?'* However, most have had a good think, have had to change their routine to attend and some will have left it until symptoms are unbearable. For those with chronic illnesses requiring check-ups, such as diabetes or hypertension, getting time off work regularly can be problematic. Many employers understand that employees require health supervision but some can make life very difficult for people, increasing the burden of long-term illness and complications. Even those who are retired and ageing can have difficulty attending, as they rely increasingly on a relative to bring them and may need to arrange appointments around their helper's time off. Next time you are frustrated that a patient on home visits has managed to get to the shops but not to the surgery, check that you have the full details; it might be that their availability is limited by factors outside their control.

Accessing the general practice

Having decided to see the GP, many patients report difficulties getting an appointment and find that getting past GP reception staff is difficult. Reception staff are often trained to ask questions about ailments in order to triage appointments with the appropriate HCP at the optimal time (optimal for the reported symptoms and practice availability, but not necessarily for the patient). This is because of the pressure general practice is experiencing in offering timely modern health care to its population, as well as the many different grades of HCP now working in GP practices. Whenever a solution to general practice pressure is created, it seems to revolve around deconstructing the patient journey so that various parts can be scrutinized and replicated by others, then a new staff role slotted in to cope with one part of it. This leaves patient care lacking full continuity and oversight.

If patients make their appointments in person at the GP reception desk their request may be audible to other patients queuing behind them. The unfortunate receptionist is commonly stuck between a patient wanting to be seen, a clinic list with no availability, and occasionally HCPs who are unhelpful when extra work is piled on, as they are at maximum capacity already. Reception staff are trained to keep patient confidentiality and usually write a few words by the patient's name on the computerised clinic list to inform the GP of the problem, e.g. 'bad cough, has asthma'.

Patients sometimes comment that paramedics, receptionists, nurses and doctors call them by their first name in every sentence and are over-familiar. This is sometimes liked but other times can cause complaints. With computerisation, it is difficult to capture individual wishes over time, as records tend to scroll into the ether. This means it can be difficult to maintain a 'front page' which might highlight patient name preferences.

Patients who do not turn up for appointments are a big issue for practices in terms of cost and time, and sometimes because of serious concerns about their health. We all have patients who have a major illness but do not like a medical model and fail to turn up despite personal reminders. Sometimes patients are homeless and it is impossible to check up on them if they don't attend. Most people, though, have just forgotten. GPs are highly organised but many people, especially if not working, do not keep a diary, might not know what day it is or the exact time. We know ourselves that after a couple of weeks on holiday we are often uncertain of the day, time, even month exactly; calendar time is no longer a motivator in our usually very regimented lives! It is a perfect clash of cultural norms when a patient doesn't arrive, having forgotten, but the practice takes a very dim view as there just isn't space to accommodate rebookings.

Telephone consultations

Some patients are not offered face-to-face appointments and some patients do not require or want them. To reduce appointments patients are sometimes offered email advice (e-consultations are being developed with AI and/or online consultations with doctors and nurses), but more commonly it's telephone consultations. Unfortunately for the GP, the ten minutes on the phone may not save time if it requires a further face-to-face consultation. Remote conversations require a specific skill set in detailed enquiry. The GP is effectively blind to nonverbal and visual examination clues and the patient is under pressure to answer possibly unexpected questions quickly and accurately. There is the possibility of misinterpretation on both sides. In addition, not meeting the patient can lead to regret if the patient's condition worsens disastrously. Statistical likelihood for given symptoms tends to assume a 'usual' set of common illnesses and courses, potentially missing rare and unusual items. Successful telephone scenarios often revolve around enquiries within a fit population or predictable discussions to protect the doctor and especially the patient. A few consultations which are very suitable for the phone are listed below:

- Low risk of underlying disease, e.g. consultation for first onset, nonrecurrent urinary tract infection in a young woman
- General non-illness information, e.g. contraception, holiday vaccinations, enquiries about time off work with diarrhoea
- Planned contact to test algorithms of care in known scenarios, e.g. response to painkillers after initial face-to-face consultation
- Triage to decide urgency and best HCP provider in the practice

Scenario: Patient not connecting symptoms with illness
Mrs X, 60 years old, attends clinic with dizziness. As is often the case, the history was vague. The GP noticed that Mrs X was winking (blepharospam) repeatedly with the right eye. When asked why, Mrs X said she had a 'bit of conjunctivitis and was using Golden Eye Ointment and not to worry about that'. On examination, the patient opened her eye briefly and with difficulty, to reveal an orbital abscess. The patient was admitted by ambulance and underwent enucleation of the eye. This was totally unexpected and rare.

The patient had not connected the eye with dizziness and this would have been impossible to diagnose without a face-to-face consultation.

Scenario: Successful planned algorithm of care by telephone
Mr Y has severe shingles pain which wakes him at night and has met his GP. He was started on a slow (modified) release tramadol tablet to offer night-time analgesia. The GP suggested that, if this did not suit or was not effective, he try the alternatives

of amitriptyline or morphine MR at night to get to sleep. Mr Y could work his way through the medications to find best pain control without returning to clinic, provided he phoned in at a set time weekly to discuss his analgesia. Written names were given so Mr Y could remember them. The phone consultation discussed effectiveness, dose, and side-effects. Mr Y could say if he wanted to persevere on current therapy or try an alternative, in which case a prescription was left at the reception desk and a clinic appointment avoided. Mr Y achieved reasonably good pain control on amitriptyline, having felt very sick on tramadol. The final phone call discussed decreasing use of medication and gave a clinic time for a pain and medication review six weeks later, face-to-face. Three consultations were saved and the less than 10-minute phone call was more convenient for both the doctor and Mr Y.

When consulting on the telephone, assume you are being recorded. In case the caller is on speaker phone, ask who is listening and consent them to hear the questions. Using speaker phone is excellent for anyone with hearing impairment, which includes most of the elderly with presbyaccussis. Once the clinician has undertaken this initial check, the telephone consultation should delve into details of history and effects of symptoms, asking questions to exclude severe illness and checking the patient has understood and agreed with the clinical decision made, including when to re-contact the practice. Frequently patients have already waited a week with symptoms before contacting their GP and may need to be examined when they phone. That said, some people do present their symptoms very early. If a patient appears unreliable, always bring them in to be seen.

Scenario: Unreliable patient

Miss X (mum): I am calling because my baby is 18 months old and has a temperature. I just want advice, I don't need to come in.

GP: Have you checked the temperature?

Miss X: Yes, it's 68°C.

GP: (further questions reveal a probably healthy baby) We would like you to bring her in to us now, as the temperature isn't accurate. Bring the thermometer with you please; let's have a look at it.

Any patient who thinks a temperature of 68°C is possible (normal limits are 36.5–37.5°C) is unreliable and anything else said may also be unreliable. In this case, the child was well and the temperature was normal. The mother was intelligent but panicking.

Telephone consultations require excellent record keeping but avoid commonly used, nondefensible phrases such as 'no red flags', which have no specific point of reference. There are telephone consultation observation tool models available through the RCGP.

I recommend including:

- Who is present in this phone call? Are they consented to listen in?
- Symptoms and timing. Is the condition worsening? What has been tried and has it helped?

- What examination findings can the individual relate by phone? How ill do they feel?
- Psychosocial exploration. Why have they phoned and why now? What is their psychosocial circumstance?
- What is their health belief?
- Discussion about diagnostic possibilities and likelihoods
- Discussion about care plan. Include specifics of follow up if required or pre-scribing advice with benefits and harms.
- Does the GP want to check on anything and when?
- What if the symptoms change? What should the person do?
- Recap to ensure the caller agrees. Have they understood what was said?
- Is there anything else they want to ask?
- Record keeping

Arrival at the practice

In many practices patients' now self-register on arrival by typing their date of birth into a computer screen or by fingerprint. The ability of reception staff to spot the patient who doesn't look well, e.g. with crushing chest pain on arrival but doesn't want to make a fuss, is lost. Once sat in the waiting room, the patient's name usually comes up on an overhead screen with the room number for the doctor. Frequently there is no anonymity. A problematic example is a young girl attending with a termination of pregnancy request. Some waiting patient, a friend or relative of her mum, could let the family know she was in the health centre ('they wouldn't have recognised her but then her name came up on the doctor's screen; hasn't she grown!') Some doctors call the patient in by name; they like the personalisation and can gather information about gait, breathlessness, pallor, cyanosis, distraction, depression, panic, happiness, swollen hand joints, etc. before the patient is even in the consulting room.

Scenario: Gait and demeanor
The GP calls a patient in at the waiting room and returns to the clinic room, wait-ing by the door. The GP notices that this 58-year-old walks unsteadily with a stick, is listing to the left, and has a poor gait. Once sat in clinic, the patient says she has come to start anticoagulation, as her hospital OPC letter directs. The GP asks whether she has had any falls and finds she is falling at least twice a week, due to an already investigated and monitored neurological condition. She had arrived at the practice by disability scooter. The consultation discusses risks and benefits of antico-agulation, and in this case both parties agreed that it was a nonstarter.

Problems with consultations: Time and money

There are several GP employment models. Almost all GPs used to have a General Medical Services (GMS) contract but some now work to a slightly higher income on a Primary Medical Services (PMS) contract. There are also GPs who do not run practices but are salaried. GP gross pay, if a practice partner (not salaried but instead a profit-sharing partner) requires tax, national insurance, practice expenses and wages, etc. to be removed before the GP collects his/her income which is a set, agreed share of the end profit. A salaried GP does not usually have as much administration and responsibility in running the practice and earns less. GPs are, on the face of it, well paid and usually have permanent work. An online net salary calculator at http://content.digital.nhs.uk/catalogue/PUB18375/gp-earn-ex-1312-rep.pdf states that the taxable income in 2014/15 for a GMS GP was £96,000 and for a PMS GP was £106,800. Salaried GPs in the UK, pre-tax, earned £54,600. The figures are difficult to make total sense of as they vary between practices, according to hours worked, and whether sickness insurance and defence subscriptions are included or not. Defence subscriptions vary but for an average full-time GP are about £7,500–£8,000 a year.

We are therefore going to take a figure of £65,000 as a take-home pay for an average full-time, five-day a week GMS/PMS GP partner working and running a practice. The NHS confederation website at http://www.nhsconfed.org/resources/key-statistics-on-the-nhs states in 2017 that there are 7,454 GP practices in England with an equivalent of 33,423 full-time GPs; 15,827 nurses in GP practices; 10,009 GP direct patient care staff; and 65,334 admin/non-clinical staff. It is difficult to track workload rates as so many GPs come in their own time to complete administrative work, preferring to be paid for less hours in clinics in order to have some work-life balance. Administrative work includes actioning test results, visits, letters, administrative forms, government-led activities and signing repeat prescriptions. GP's have varying hours of work in clinics but also telephone consultation. Recently a GP complained that 80 test results arrived for him to action in three days and this is not unusual. We will explore how this may affect decision making in the 'revolving test door' section later on.

The number of female GPs is now over 50%. If they become mothers they may take maternity leave and while children are young many female GPs will work part-time hours to facilitate child care. Male GPs may also need flexibility for child care. The old patriarchal model of a 'full-time qualification-to-grave GP' is no more. GPs of both sexes are more likely to want a portfolio role with flexible hours. This clearly has implications on the number of GPs available to see patients at any given time.

There is also a tension between wanting to see more patients and earn more and being chronically overworked. On a quiet day, GPs may see 30 patients in clinic, split into two surgeries of 15, plus two visits and administration. That is 32 patients a day over five days (160 patient clinic or visit contacts a week) and assuming a £65,000 take home pay for a 46-week year (6 weeks of holidays or study leave), this amounts to approximately £8.80 payment per patient seen. This does not include recompense for telephone consultations or administrative work. GP workload is not linear and it is almost unheard of to have a quiet day. Many GPs see many more patients than the example above.

Below is a model day. It is very approximate but gives the reader some insight. It is clear that there is no slack and no time to be creative about the direction of the GP's role. There is no space for emergencies, long discussions, managing queries or complaints. Any of these problems stretch available time, or the GP often cuts down their hours and income to accommodate them, but this further reduces society's health care provision in terms of numbers of people seen.

Model day:

8.00 am–8.30 am: urgent test results

8.30 am–11.00 am: 15 patients at 10 minutes a consultation

11.15 am: Problems from staff, test result reading with actions, hospital letters, administrative forms, referral letters, prescriptions, practice meetings

1.30 pm–2.30 pm: two visits

3.00 pm–5.30 pm: 15 patients at 10 minutes a consultation. Added phone calls and administration.

There may be extra patients slotted in the day. Some practices share all urgent and non-urgent cases out and some have an 'on-call' GP each day who will see the urgent cases.

This is a conservative estimate as stated above, and these figures are not easy to find via an online search. However, reports showing that the workload of GPs has climbed over the last decade are common, despite GPs no longer providing out of hours (OOHs) work in evenings and weekends as part of their contract and delegating more of their traditional role to other HCPs. The day above may seem manageable but every week, month, and year after year it is hard work. GPs work 8.00 am–6.30 pm as an average contracted day, though there are extended hour schemes with the government. For many there is a temptation to see more patients faster, squeeze consultation skills, and earn more. The drivers for skipping professional consultation skills to increase income are one of the challenges faced by general practice.

Patients want a GP with lots of time. GPs want time to act to high standards, but the cost to society and governments would be high if they were to be paid 'fairly'. If the consultation becomes an obstruction to getting through the day and receiving a monthly pay check, then patients become an inconvenience to the job.

Scenario: One of the fastest consultations ever related

Mr Y: I have come to see you because the other GP this morning gave me this (hands over an uncashed prescription with amoxicillin prescribed on it)

GP: What's wrong with this?

Mr Y: I told the doctor that I have felt tired and weepy for two weeks and I am worried about why that is. The GP didn't even look at me but handed me this prescription and said it was due to influenza. I was in and out before I could sit down. I'm sure that's not right.

GP: Okay, I understand your complaint. Please start again, I am listening. Tell me what's happening....

Analysis of patients experience above:

- Lack of any sort of consultation for Mr Y.
- Secondary poor reputation develops for the first GP. Mr Y has a poor view of the practice. Mr Y's friends and family hear this poor view.
- The poor GP performance requires someone to talk to the GP about this and to the practice manager. There is a need to investigate the GP's performance in other areas and at other times to check competency.

- An inappropriate prescription of a penicillin antibiotic on many counts. Antibiotics are not indicated in depression and are not indicated for a viral illness, like influenza. There are inappropriate drug and dispensing costs to society and the practice develops poor metrics for the GP prescribing audits by national bodies. Inappropriate antibiotics, if Mr Y takes them, promotes antibiotic resistance, possible patient side-effects without benefit, and sends the message to Mr Y that antibiotics cure all ills when they don't.
- Time and NHS costs accrue in needing a second GP consultation and actioning the above items.

Working at capacity with no slack means that colleague holidays, HCP illness, unexpected or unscheduled work, or a patient complaint (genuine or otherwise) can tip the balance for doctors from caring professionals to stressed, anxious people who aren't coping. GPs also develop physical illnesses, such as coughs or nausea, or may ignore a more serious illness and continue at work because of the pressure the practice is under. The GP may be fit, quick, and young or may be older, slower, with some stiffness and osteoarthritis (OA), with aching wrists and knees.

The GP under strain may reduce his/her hours and go part-time, spending a day unpaid completing practice paper work. The GP who can retire may leave early (on a reduced pension) and that doctor's clinical skills are then removed from the health care system for good. These are currently common scenarios. There is little job satisfaction in having an unmanageable workload.

On locum work: Some GPs solve their practice problems by leaving partnership or salaried appointments and working as locums to achieve more control or flexibility of their workload. Indeed, many newly qualified GPs do not enter partnership but prefer locum work from the outset. There is no shortage of locum work presently, especially with the current model of GPs working some of their sessions at CCGs to lead on area health improvements. Locums are paid for a pre-agreed workload based on the number of patients (usually 12 or 15 in a clinic and sometimes visits and administration). Locums are self-employed and most find it convenient to employ an accountant to address issues such as National Insurance contributions, pension contributions, tax liability, and tax deductible expenses such as defence subscriptions and medical subscriptions, e.g. membership of the Royal College of General Practitioners (RCGP) and medical equipment. Being a locum can be rewarding as GPs can work when they wish, with a lot less paper work and administration. They can opt to visit patients, or not, and set their own charges within a competitive market for their rates of pay. They are paid pro rata more than a partner for seeing each patient. If they don't like a surgery they don't have to go back and they are less likely to follow up patient care. Some locums may work for many months full-time, often covering a doctor's maternity leave and get a taste of partnership practice whereas others prefer to have less continuity. Their case load is more likely to be acute illnesses. Some locums in early year careers like to work hard for a number of months and then travel the world.

The downsides of being a locum are that they pay higher defence subscriptions and must make their own provisions for sick pay, holiday pay and maternity pay. There is no death in service benefit and they must invoice and chase up payments. They may need to master a number of computer and referral systems across geographical areas and there is less support from colleagues. It can be difficult to get feedback on patient care from colleagues for annual mandatory appraisals. There is also the lack of continuity of care.

Scenario: A patient appreciates continuity
A young woman attends a GP and towards the end of the consultation says 'I asked to see you because I remember when my mum was very ill with cancer some years ago you visited, called an ambulance and waited with her. I went downstairs to watch for the ambulance and she told me that you sat next to her on the bed, holding her hand and had a lovely chat'.

Why have a consultation?

There are several reasons why GPs are consulted and they can be divided into four main groups (although, as GPs have open access, any reason is valid):

1. **To discuss symptoms in order to diagnose or to exclude illness**, especially serious illnesses like cancers. These are new acute consultations.
    This is very important. GPs are different to secondary care doctors, who have usually had patients triaged and prediagnosed via primary care before they meet them. For GPs the question, 'Is this patient safe to go home?'means that we look for disease but we also look for normality. We may use tests to confirm normality rather than disease. An example would be a normal CA125 in a woman with normal examination findings but complaining of some abdominal distension. In this case a low CA125 makes ovarian cancer highly unlikely.
2. **To support people with illnesses in body, psychological and social terms.**
3. **To screen people for illnesses which early on may have no symptoms** (such as type 2 diabetes, T2DM) and **to screen people for their likelihood of developing future illnesses**, such as coronary heart disease (CHD) or stroke (cerebrovascular accident, CVA) caused by factors such as hypertension or high cholesterol, as patients cannot measure or interpret these easily themselves. This requires tests, decisions and patient communication which can be time-consuming if not done well. We talk further about this below to help the reader avoid related pitfalls of practice.
4. **To medically monitor patients with known illnesses to keep them as well as possible** and prevent, if possible, future worsening of their condition. This includes monitoring medication which, as patients age and collect illnesses, increases and with which the body may be less able to cope. Monitoring conditions and illnesses is not the same as support in the second point above – monitoring here is all medical.

There are many more reasons but these four reasons to consult are the most common. The clinician will use different skills depending on the consultation type.

Bringing patients back: Avoiding the revolving test door

A fair proportion of consultations are due to GP-instigated requests and we should ask the followng:

- How useful is this consultation request?
- How necessary is it?
- How does the patient fit into the doctor initiated request to attend?

Consider a patient who has had a consultation and a test; perhaps during a new patient check or a well-person check. The test might be to monitor a chronic condition (like diabetes) or a test for medication suitability, e.g. checking potassium and renal function in a patient taking an angiotensin converting enzyme inhibitor (ACEI), e.g. ramipril. Perhaps the test arrived as a check to exclude a condition or illness, e.g. a thyroid function test in someone complaining of lethargy and weight gain.

The patient may have had the test done by any of a variety of HCPs; the assistant practitioner (AP), practice nurse, nurse practitioner, health physician associate, GP locum, GP partner, maybe even the GP actioning the blood test result. The test may be sent through from the hospital after an inpatient stay or after a OPC visit. Either way the GP logs on to action the day's blood tests. It is time-consuming, clicking into the patient's notes to find the relevant entries, uncover why the test was done, and create a logical, accurate action. Pragmatically, the GP needs to get on and action the results list. The next clinic or visit is waiting. Unfortunately, the GP may press from a drop-down list of actions (and scores of GPs have reported to me that they have done this) 'see patient non-urgent' or occasionally 'see patient urgent'.

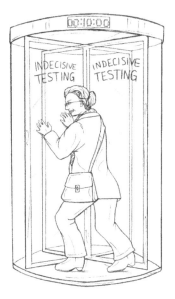

The revolving test door.

A practice receptionist actions the messages from the GP results and is tasked with phoning the patient, or dropping them a standard letter to ask him/her to come into the practice to discuss their blood test results.

Scenario: Diagnosing Type 2 diabetes (T2DM) from a HbA1c

A glycosylated haemoglobin blood test (HbA1c) measures how much glucose is attached to circulating blood cells over many weeks. This is raised in type 2 and type 1 diabetics (T2DM and T1IDDM) and can be used to guide diabetes diagnoses, providing there are no haemoglobin problems so that the blood count remains constant over weeks. HbA1c is also used to measure diabetic disease control in known diabetic patients. HbA1c has had a change in its units so that people with long-standing diabetes have two sets of indices to compare, their old and their newer units. A HbA1c conversion table can be useful, as older patients may still think in older unit (this was as a percentage) terms. Prior to using HbA1c as a diagnostic test, clinicians made the diagnosis of diabetes by

- Random blood sugar with symptoms
- Fasting blood glucose
- Glucose tolerance test

These tests are still valid.

In addition, obstetricians diagnosing diabetes in pregnancy use a glucose tolerance test (haemoglobin varies in pregnancy, making HbA1c less reliable as a diagnostic test for diabetes in pregnant individuals). To make life more complicated, obstetricians use different glucose levels for diagnosis (lower) than in non-pregnant individuals having a glucose tolerance test. Changing behaviour is very difficult if a clinician has acquired a system or knowledge that works for him/her. It is not surprising then that this area has created some clinician confusion.

In T2DM the patient may run low on insulin from the pancreas and/or may have resistance to the action of insulin at peripheral sites, related often to obesity. Insulin resistance occurs in almost all T2DM diabetics. There is often a family history of T2DM and it is a common condition of older age groups. Unlike the T1IDDMs, who require insulin to live, the T2DM group can often manage with diet, weight loss and tablets. However, T2DM is a serious condition as diabetic complications, affecting the patient's circulation, nervous system, kidneys and vision can lead to disability and death. Diagnosing and monitoring T2DM to improve the patient's outlook is important. It is a very common condition but is largely a biochemical condition with few symptoms and so understanding that biochemical testing is imperative to assessing control and outcomes is important. The World Health Organisation (WHO) states that a HbA1c of below 42 mmol/L is unlikely to be diabetes and a HbA1c over 48 mmol/L is likely to mean diabetes. There are exceptions of course. The volume of HbA1c tests appearing in a GP inbox is large, and remember, they may relate to known diabetic monitoring or to tests to diagnose diabetes. Back to the scenario:

A GP sees a HbA1c test of 48 mmoml/L. He is short of time and there is a long list of tests to action. There is a response 'action list' and a free text box, so the GP clicks the 'see GP non-urgent' box. The GP doesn't know if this patient has had a screening test for diabetes, if it is a follow up test, or if the test is monitoring a known diabetic. There is no time to access the notes and check. To click into the notes, search for the reason for testing, and find out when and who arranged it takes some time and patients are waiting to be seen and time is ticking on. In this case, the patient was a newly diagnosed diabetic patient and ideally would have had the test repeated and been referred to the diabetic practice lead. Instead the patient was called into the practice, met a GP who was not the diabetic lead and had not seen the test or patient before. This GP explained the diagnosis and referred the patient to the diabetic practice lead. The patient was annoyed to need another appointment, having rushed in, believing himself to be seriously ill and had taken time off work. This wasted, in effect, one consultation for the GP, the patient, and the practice. He still needed a second confirmatory test before the diagnosis could be made and ended up attending twice more. This can become a revolving door.

Despite time issues it would have ultimately been quicker (and cheaper to the NHS) when actioning the test result to ask:

- What is the problem?
- What should I do if I am not sure?
- What action do I want to take?
- What is the best way of taking this action?
- What does the patient need to know and how do they feel?
- How am I going to communicate with the patient and other practice team members?
- What is the time frame for this?
- Is this the most efficient patient-centered care?

Other commonly misinterpreted, incompletely or incorrectly actioned test results which cause patients to enter the revolving, indecisive test door are renal functions (electronic glomerular filtration rate [eGFR]), cholesterols, and minor abnormal full blood count (FBC) tests. Patients from differing UK regions have related being asked to return to practices, including rushing to the GP thinking they have leukaemia, because they are told their blood test is 'abnormal' only to find that the abnormality is 'normal for them' or requires investigation but is non-urgent with no clinical sequalae at that time. No one wants to miss a severe test abnormality, but lesser abnormalities, some of which are not abnormal for that patient, should not create patient anxiety. Being clear about guidelines, diagnoses, action plans, and, as always, good communication are required to provide excellent practice. This requires time. We will rotate through the test door again and again in this book.

Consultation models

There are several consultation models and GPs may choose one or combine models. The skills of good consulting lie in using our senses, especially our ears. The GP facilitates people into making the best decisions at that time about their own care. To do this, we use our specialist knowledge of medical law and our ethical training as well as self-awareness of our own views, our best knowledge of medicine as it is known at that time, and our consultation skills. This book is divided into those sections.

Before the patient is seen. Gain as much information as possible about him/her in as short a space of time as possible. Check the patient's computerised notes for the last consultation, the last consultation with yourself, the last acute prescription, and then look at their repeat medications which reveal likely ongoing conditions or diseases. Look at the PMH screen so you may (or may not) develop some opinion as to why they are attending and any underlying issues. Their age also dictates likely illnesses.

Ensure you have a comfortable workstation. Some GPs complain of neck and back pain due to reaching to the floor to turn on computers, loading paper, and swinging round to collect prescriptions or forms from the printer. The patient should be sat so that you have direct eye contact and are not sat twisted all day between patient and computer screen. Then call the patient in.

Running Late. If you have a problem, like running late, apologise immediately to reduce the patient's frustration and allow him/her to move onto why they have attended. Work out a couple of helpful phrases, such as 'Thank you very much for waiting for me; I am running late'. The patient usually responds with an understanding smile and is pleased to have been thanked. The angry patient usually exhales their rage and states why the wait has irritated them. This gives the GP an opportunity to apologise again and perhaps explain 'an earlier urgent patient problem' or that a problem 'took more time than expected', though none of us can ever state any details about any of our patients to anyone else.

Sitting down and getting the start right. Once the patient is sitting, recheck their details and introduce yourself clearly.

Sensory impairment. Assume all patients are a little hard of hearing and speak clearly and directly. Many patients are in an age group where they have presbyaccussis and presbyopia. If the patient is obviously struggling to hear, this can be an opportunity to discuss hearing aids. Many elderly people have difficulty remembering information, so check their understanding at the end of the consultation and offer a written synopsis of management plans. For anyone with severe deafness, written consultations are more reliable and allow the patient to take the conversation away to share with loved ones.

Scenario: Deafness

It had become apparent that the patient wasn't hearing well.

GP: *You are a bit hard of hearing. Have you got a hearing aid?*

Mr Y: *No, I don't want one of those.*

GP: *Are you hearing the telephone and door? May I look to see if there is any wax?*

Mr Y: *Yes, please (there was none)*

GP: *The ear canals are clear. There is no wax.*

Mr Y: *I don't want to be mucking about with a hearing aid.*

GP: *Okay, you can always come back. But do you catch what your family say when they are round? Do you get their jokes, or are they starting to not bother 'cos they have to repeat the punch line? They will end up talking to you on a need to know basis you know!*

Mr Y: *You're right, better get me one then, please.*

Hearing impairment is helped by improvements in speaker phone technology and volume control. Using video means that some individuals can also lip-read remote consultations. Some remote consultation apps use typeset so that hearing loss is immaterial.

Visual impairment is also very common in our elderly, e.g. age related macular degeneration (ARMD), and this can also be helped by smart phones, e-notebooks or laptops. The ability to provide good contrast and lighting on-screen, with increases in typeset size, has helped many visually-impaired people. They may need to consult a younger relative to skill up. If there is no one available Age UK will often help. If vision is very poor, using a smart phone or computer to provide auditory interpretation of text is helpful.

Once the elderly have difficulty going outside due to mobility problems, dementia, or are staying in as carers, social media can be a wonderful way for them to stay in touch with old friends. It surprises me how many elderly can take on information technology (IT) skills easily and enjoy them.

On aggression. Aggression is often due to intense anxiety, unless someone is under the influence of alcohol or drugs, or seriously mentally ill. There are a few patients, often well-known offenders in a practice, who are difficult due to aggression. Some people cannot control anger and have anxiety on top of intrinsic personality traits, developmental experiences, or current anxiety-provoking issues. Some are used to, and so anticipate, rejection.

Scenario: Expecting rejection

The patient attends the desk shouting at the receptionist
'I want an appointment now or get the f***ing doctor to visit'.
The receptionist is shocked and relates it to the GP. When the patient is confronted about the behavior by the GP at the end of the consultation she is apologetic and ashamed.
It is likely that the patient expected not to be seen and, being anxious over their condition, came shouting about rejection before asking politely.

If aggressive behaviour doesn't settle down, let the person know that they are making you tense. Often the patient will look surprised, as he or she has not really noticed it themselves, or reflected on how it feels for the GP. They may then settle down and the ensuing consultation runs smoothly.

Scenario: An aggressive patient

Miss X: *I've waited four days for this appointment. It's f***ing disgusting.*

GP: Thank you for waiting; I'm Dr X, you are here now. What can I do for you?
Miss X (angry): I want the results of my X-ray and something f***ing done about it now.
GP: Can you speak a little slower please; you're making me feel anxious.
Miss X: Oh, sorry, doctor, yes of course….

So, people can behave inappropriately if anxious to be seen, expecting rejection, or are worried about themselves. Their worry may not be in the medical aspect of their lives. GPs should support the reception staff and colleagues against aggression. The examples above explore unintended aggression which has over spilt.

Another group who are aggressive however are committed to aggression and some may be 'mind altered'. Rarely, they might have a psychotic mental illness but most of this group are on drugs or drunk. I strongly advise GPs not to get involved with this group at that time. My advice is to close down the consultation and get help. There should be an alarm call button on work computer screens or desks if there are problems which need staff help. Occasionally the police will need to be called. Never forget that patients who are violent, uncontrollable and leave you unable to manage their care, or to care for those patients waiting patiently in the waiting room after them, can be seen in a commissioned clinic. There are GP practices trained to deal specifically with aggressive patients, sometimes at a police station.

The first sentence you utter to your patient sets yourself up as the doctor.

Some GPs say, 'How can I help you?' The 'I' places them in a helpful, in-charge role.

Some GPs say, 'What is the problem?'

I am not too precious about this as patients appreciate that the conversation has to kick off with some colloquial phrase.

A neutral start is, 'Hello, I am Dr X, are you…..?'. The patient then starts the conversation.

If busy, some GPs use, 'What problem can I help you with today?' The GP is signaling that the patient needs to be focused. A common response might be, 'Well, it's a couple of things, actually doctor'. In this case the patient has heard the message the GP has sent them and settled on two items, there might have been more.

It is up to ourselves as clinicians to choose the best opener for our patient, our self, and our waiting patients.

The Laws and regulations section of this book discusses capacity and consent. It is important to check that the patient consents, and that you offer a chaperone, for any examination which might be construed as intimate by them. They should have capacity to understand the consultation. This may require a translator, large text, or writing the consultation down between you.

Patients will choose the consultation style and doctor that suits their problem. If the problem is not urgent and the patient has lived in the area long enough to be a part of the community, they often ask friends and family for opinions about the local GP practice and select the GP who suits their problem. If a patient wants a longer talk about their problem or more than one issue, a mental health problem for example, they select a GP who their neighbours tell them will provide time and empathy, but a GP who might run late. If a patient wants to be in and out with a quick issue they will select a GP who is more time-efficient. As GPs, we develop a suite of consultation styles dependent on the patient and their problems. In addition, it's not always helpful to continually bring up past issues to patients. For example, if I told my GP about my grief this may become the problem that defines me to that GP. I would not want to be reminded about it every time I went, in a misplaced use of connection and empathy, when I have closed that problem and moved on. Be led by the patient, sensitive to their verbal and nonverbal signals, but also let them develop as complete individuals: our knowledge of them is a small piece of their lives.

History taking–data collection. The next step is to uncover the reason for the patient's attendance. It may be a simple, obvious problem or, more usually, requires the patient to give a narrative of the issues which we are trained to interpret in a medical manner. I use the word medical in a psychological and social framework that covers all aspects of health. Using the inner question, 'Why have they come *now*?', is very useful. Often a condition worsened, e.g. increasing pain, perhaps disturbing their sleep, or a family member has encouraged them to attend.

Scenario: Continuing pain

Mr Y, 63 years old, developed an inflammatory arthritis over two weeks and couldn't bring his fingers to his palms to make a fist. He also had tender, swollen wrists and was referred to rheumatology and started on therapy. He visited his GP three times in the year with severe pain and stiffness and the GP also visited him twice when he couldn't get out of bed easily. The GP felt his disease was poorly controlled by hospital colleagues; he was always immobile and in pain. One day the GP asked him why he had come on that particular day and he said, 'I don't know why it's today, doctor, but it occasionally just flares up. I had a great walking holiday two weeks ago, you wouldn't believe the change. I was managing Lake District fells.' This man functioned very well over 90% of the time; a man who the GP had assumed had a chronic debilitating disease. He was generally happy with his disease management.

Listen to the patient's explanation of why they have attended and uncover the history and facts about the problems, their aetiology and the effects on the patient. Use nonverbal behaviour and listening skills to encourage the patient to tell their story. This is their narrative and after a couple of minutes most patients have told you a history which would take ten minutes to find out in small disjointed pieces had we interrogated them. Even obsessive patients tend to be finished by three minutes. There are of course some patients who just don't stop, and you must retain control of the consultation and interject if required. Stating '*I am going to stop you there and I am going to summarise what you have said before we move on*' is a way of halting the flow. Patients have described GPs using their hands like traffic signals to stop them and move them on. Whilst this is not best practice, some people contextualize their problems by telling their GPs exactly what they were doing at every step of the way, and this can take a long time! After hearing the patient's history, ask questions to outline associated features, exclude other illnesses, exclude or include serious symptoms, and then deliver a synopsis back to the patient so you both agree on the problem. These are closed, focused questions. Establish how the patient is functioning compared to their normal baseline health. It is surprising how many patients will not relate that they wake with pain until asked.

If someone tells, or hints, at something uncomfortable to hear, the GP has a professional responsibility to unravel it. A common example would be that an elderly demented man *'is not eating much this last few days'*. This is easily passed over, but he may only be getting a cup of soup a day.

Scenario: Unexpected facts
Mr Y has severe sciatica and attends his GP. The GP takes an excellent history of back pain and sciatica and asks what the patient has taken so far. He has taken paracetamol. The GP asks how many and he has taken 14 that day because they aren't effective for his pain. This patient may be at risk of a paracetamol overdose and related liver failure. He was annoyed to be referred into hospital but was treated with N-acetyl cysteine, the antidote for paracetamol overdose, to prevent liver failure and grateful afterwards.

We call noticing and hearing non-obvious consultation items 'cues', and clinicians have a duty to acknowledge inwardly that a patient looks in pain, ill, thin, obese, shy, depressed. These patients may drop in messages such as the following:

A woman requesting contraception: *'I've never had any children'*.

A mother over her daughter: *'I don't think her vaginal itching is due to any abuse or anything'*.

A depressed looking patient who quietly says, *'It doesn't matter'*.

Watch, listen and pick up patient cues and associated messages.

In the consultation, there are three commonly used clinician techniques:

Facilitation is the GP's own nonverbal or sound-based communication to facilitate the patient. This shows listening and might include sitting forward, making eye contact, head nodding, mumbling, 'Yes, I see', etc. We remember when our

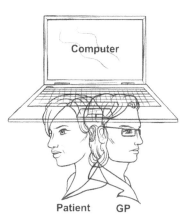

The modern consultation triad.

hand might occasionally touch the hand of someone in tears as an act of professional and human empathy. Nowadays our hand is on the mouse, our eyes are averted from the patient to the computer screen, and we have to make a conscious effort to communicate as a human being and not as part of an artificial intelligence system. Avoid a system with intelligence but without humanity.

Reflection may be repeating something the patient has said in order to invite them to expand upon it or it may be reflecting a mood or unspoken observation. Examples of reflection to match the patient's statement and invite expansion:

To the woman asking for contraception: *'You said you've never had any children, what are you thinking?'*

To the mother over her daughter: *'You said you don't think her vaginal itching is due to any abuse or anything, are you worried about that?'*

To the depressed looking patient: *'You said it doesn't matter; what doesn't matter and why?'*

This too is the absorption of the patient's manner and speech in tone and cadence, and it may be appropriate to reflect this back. So, it would be inappropriate to speak loudly to a patient whispering due to shyness or depression, and inappropriate to whisper to a patient speaking loudly due to anxiety or deafness.

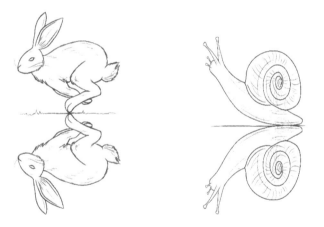

Reflecting speech and unspoken messages.

Refraction allows GPs to screen information and convey questions and messages in a way that makes sense to patients at that time. The information we receive from the patient is absorbed, as through a prism. Some may be reflected but other information undergoes bending and selection. The clinician within us uses refraction as a device to sieve out information and focus the consultation.

An example might be developing a timeline from a patient, e.g. over a period problem. Most women are not regimented over menstrual diaries, e.g. Miss X says her periods are irregular and that her last menstrual period was 'before her birthday'. The GP draws out the important information dates on paper and notes the dates of her menstrual cycle, when she last had intercourse, when the worrying bleeding began, etc. to narrow down the information. The patient can then see the information in medical terms and understand it.

Conditions in which symptoms have waxed and waned, or when different medications have been prescribed over months, drawn out like this can be helpful. You are both literally on the same page.

That said, refraction is usually verbal. For example, a patient attends with irritable bowel syndrome (IBS) but on history taking, reveals an alcohol intake amounting to alcoholism. The GP focuses the questions to alcohol-related problems and includes questions about work and relationships. In leaving the IBS symptoms and refracting information and focusing, the patient admits to problems with alcohol affecting his life and creating anxiety. It dawns on the patient that alcohol is a major factor in his presentation, but he hadn't realised it. The GP has absorbed the patient's information and focused the questions to explore and achieve a specific outcome.

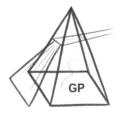

Refraction to convey focus.

After data collection, check the facts with the patient; are you accurate so far?

Next ask the patient whether they have any ideas or concerns about the symptoms or expectations for the consultation.

Scenario: A common cough
Mr Y, 80 years old, attends with a two-week history of a cough. It is dry, he doesn't cough in clinic, nor at night, it appears not to be much of a problem. Having gathered the history and examined him the GP is unsure why he has come. He doesn't appear ill.

GP: *What do you think the problem is? Are you thinking you need antibiotics?*
Mr Y: *No I don't think they will work. I just want something to stop the cough.*

As cough suppressants aren't effective evidence-based therapies and may make him dopey, e.g. codeine cough linctus, he might as well take a warm cordial or suck a boiled sweet instead of attending his GP. Consequently, he was offered no treatment. He was reassured and safety netted to return if the cough hadn't gone in another two weeks. He was satisfied and said had simply come for a check-up because he lived alone.

The next phase of the consultation is to check for any other problems and how patients are getting on with relevant continuing health problems. Ask about risk factors and people's social and psychological circumstances, if relevant. Check the medication screens, acute and chronic medications with them, and any allergies to medications. Now you are beginning to think about management, medication and illness interactions.

Examination

It is possible to examine patients whilst collecting the history data. Examinations may get us off our chairs and keeps us fresh and more alert, rather than slumping over the computer as the clinic progresses. GPs use skills and, like centuries of clinicians before us, detect illnesses with their hands.

Firstly, put the patient into an 'acutely seriously ill' or 'not acutely seriously ill' bucket by checking vital signs. They rarely let us down. Think about what your minimum examination set is in your clinic. Do you want a peak flow meter, pulse oximeter, different blood pressure cuff sizes, thermometers, tape measure, weighing scales, torch, opthalmoscope, otoscope and stethoscope with you? Have you got gloves and speculums if wanted? Are there in date urinalysis sticks, a spirometer, and a capillary glucose meter around if you want them? Do you want access to a fetal sonicaid? Is the emergency station available and familiar to you? Make definite decisions about your examination kit and ensure it is available for you routinely. This relates to our defined skill set which is discussed further later on.

There are four sorts of examination frameworks that GPs use when thinking about patients: diagnosing normal signs, diagnosing 'not-normal' signs, expecting abnormal examination findings (targeted examination) and continuing symptoms and negative examination findings.

DIAGNOSING NORMAL SIGNS

Examinations are great for confirming normality, if that is the GP diagnosis. This is important because in primary care if we believe the patient to be normal then we want to let them go home to their lives. To prove normality, we must detect normal examination findings. This is especially true in obstetric and paediatric examinations. Paediatric patients are often too young to give reliable histories and their illness may change quickly so it is important to give a quick head to toe examination of children.

Scenario: 3-year-old with a sore ear
Examine the child with a sore ear for temperature, rash and neck stiffness. If these develop and the child develops meningitis or sepsis then the GP must know they did their best at the time of consultation. In addition, parents may always wonder whether the signs were present at the time of consultation, waiting to be picked up. Negative findings allow the child to go home more safely, with safety netting (see below).

DIAGNOSING 'NOT-NORMAL' SIGNS

Because GPs are excellent at diagnosing normality but cannot know everything, we all make some interesting, unusual diagnoses over the years through recognising 'not-normal' signs rather than knowing the abnormality.

Scenario: 'Not-normal' ear drum
Mr Y, 40 years old, complained of right-sided deafness. Examination of the right ear revealed a small red spot on the ear drum. He was referred to the ear, nose and throat (ENT) clinic for the abnormal appearance with the words 'it looks like a cherry on the ear drum, please can you check it'. He had a cherry haemangioma, subsequently removed.

Scenario: 'Not-normal' wrist swelling
Mrs X, 60 years old, attends her GP with a 'varicose vein' over her dorsal wrist. The GP felt a smallish swelling but not a typical varicose vein, and not a typical ganglion. On referral and investigation, it was a leiomyosarcoma and the arm was amputated.

GPs frequently pick up opportune skin cancers such as squamous cell cancers and malignant melanomas by keeping their eyes open when examining chests and abdomens. Basal cell skin cancer is especially common.

EXPECTING ABNORMAL EXAMINATION FINDINGS – TARGETED EXAMINATION

Examination findings are very useful in confirming or diagnosing disease if there are positive findings.

Scenario: Lymphadenopathy expected to confirm lymphoma
Mr Y has lost weight recently and wakes at night with sweats which are so bad he changes beds and goes into the spare room part way through the night. There is no history of foreign travel. On examination, he has a normal temperature and two large firm lymph nodes in the right axilla. He is not jaundiced, not anaemic, and has no enlarged liver or spleen. The lymph nodes suggest a lymphoma, which was confirmed by his secondary care specialist.

Scenario: I think I have a cancer down below
Mrs X, 72 years old, thinks she has cancer 'down there' because she can feel a lump. The GP takes a history and prepares for PV and speculum. On examination, the abdomen is normal and there was a small cystocele (a prolapse of the anterior vaginal wall, common in older women) which did not require more than pelvic floor exercises, explanation and advice.

CONTINUING SYMPTOMS AND NEGATIVE EXAMINATION FINDINGS

There are groups of patents with symptoms and negative examination findings, but a significant possibility of disease, often related to their probability of disease due to age. These patients are problematic and may undergo numerous investigations with uncertain outcomes.

A common example is chronic abdominal pain, unresponsive to therapy. The pain may be a new pain or a chronic pain; it may be an exacerbation of a chronic pain; it may be the chronic pain unaltered but not alleviated. Patients may attend frequently for support. The search for effective therapy for several undiagnosed conditions and the decision of when to reexamine, reinvestigate, or re-refer the patient is problematic for all clinicians.

Doctors talk about 'negative examination findings' but there are no negative examination findings. Examinations reveal normal examination or abnormal examination findings and normal examination findings may suggest functioning organs: all very important.

Investigations

Investigations should be thought through and we have touched on this in the revolving door comments above. Tests are discussed in the knowledge and evidence section, so it is sufficient here to suggest that GPs ask themselves:

- What do I want to test for?
- What will I do with the result?

Some investigations are urgent and need to be well communicated to patients and practice staff.

Scenario: Sore throat on carbimazole
A 28-year-old woman taking carbimazole for hyperthyroidism develops a mild sore throat. In this situation, she has been told to stop the carbimazole and see the GP if concerned that day. If she feels well and does not want to see the GP she knows she should still have a full blood count (FBC) that day with the result phoned back to her later to reliably inform her of the result and any action. Actions might be admission for carbimazole drug-induced neutropenia or might be reassurance that the FBC is normal and this is not a drug-induced sore throat. The practice requires careful systems and communication to achieve this.

Talking about possibilities; probable diagnosis and management plans. At this stage, give the patient information, including normal findings, so that they can follow the GP's train of thought. Some investigations and referrals are done to follow national guidance, often to exclude a remote but important possibility of life-threatening disease, e.g. cancer. The patient may have their own views on causation and progression of an illness but usually are pleased to follow a logical management plan.

Non-drug therapy improves or cures many illnesses, which revolve around lack of body fitness, a need to relax and a need to develop an inner calm. People should understand that our bodies are 200,000 years old and change slowly. Conversely, our minds are highly adaptable. This is the conundrum of modern life: forgetting to keep in touch with the ancestral body. It can be difficult to change behaviour but people appreciate the opportunity to have control of their health.

Medical plans requiring medication or referrals, etc. require detailed instructions and explanation. Patients may stop antihypertensive lifelong medications because they think it is just a month's course. Conversely, they may continue on a medication when it is no longer required, e.g. ibuprofen for an inflamed joint when the inflammation has gone.

In deciding the management plan, the GP should use knowledge from the patient's history and examination, distill this with knowledge from current evidence-based medicine, consider laws and regulations which will influence management, and weigh up the ethics of the situation, the benefits and harms of the suggested management. GPs should discuss the latter with the patient and then let them use their autonomy so that they can make best decisions for themselves. That is the essence of excellence in general practice.

Rounding off the consultation

Rounding off the consultation requires consideration of

- What is the worst that can happen?

This is so that patients who do not follow the expected illness or recovery course know when to return, or any other action to take. This part of the consultation also includes checking the patient understands the plan and is happy to follow it. Decisions about whether the patient needs to be seen again, when, and by whom are made at the close of the consultation.

The Inner Consultation

The Inner Consultation by Dr Roger Neighbour is a great book which I highly recommend. It is applicable to any GP and HCP and is an engaging, thoughtful journey through the consultation. Within it is a detailed discussion about skill development and self-awareness for doctors in creating excellence. This excellence is centered on high-standard consulting skills and, for that brief consultation time, understanding the patient's needs in consulting, and looking forward in creating an action plan. Dr Neighbour divides the consultation into three skill sections:

1. Deciding what goal you (the GP) would like to achieve (now and in the longer term)
2. Developing skills to create a managed patient-centred consultation
3. Bringing yourself together to achieve self-worth and good performance

Dr Neighbour describes the GP as having an organizational head: this is the managerial, logical, trained processor inside us. As we all know, sat next to the organizational head are the emotional responses that we experience within consultations, that is, the instinctive feeling head. This second head encourages self-awareness, intuition, and responses that may improve the consultation.

He describes five 'checkpoints' within the consultation, to be reached in sequence, as described in the following sections.

1. **Connecting:** Establish a rapport so that the patient feels ready to disclose their symptoms or problems without holding back. During this phase, the clinician's skills include listening, asking non-leading questions, and then asking directed questions to gather data. Bringing together all verbal and non-verbal observations, the GP then creates several diagnostic hypotheses.

Dr Neighbour suggests that by skillful eliciting of information we can enter the patient's world briefly and there are no rules or proformas for this. This moves the consultation beyond the myriad of medical history templates, used in many undergraduate and hospital settings. Think and be receptive. He suggests that 'whatever works does'. The book is not 'shackling by history taking!' It is about skill building.

2. **Summarising:** Check that the clinician's data collection is accurate by summarising the patient's story and check that nothing has been missed or that a different topic does not need to be additionally discussed. At this stage, the physician will likely examine the patient and start to create an inner management plan based on likely diagnoses.

3. **Handover:** Make sure that the patient is engaged in developing the management plan and is happy to take ownership of it. Patients bring their own values and life positions with them. In this way, doctor and patient agree an outcome in the short and long-term. In giving information, it may be helpful to use the timing and vocabulary that the patient uses to meet them part way in understanding the medical problem.

4. **Safety net:** Think ahead and safeguard the patient against unexpected developments, such as worsening symptoms or failure to respond to treatment. Ensure that patients understand when to feel that the illness or condition has not run in an orderly manner, when there might be a serious risk to health, and what action to take. This is the 'what if' part of the consultation.

5. **Housekeeping:** Make sure the clinician is fit for the next patient and that you are enjoying your general practice. This might mean getting up and walking off for a cup of tea after a difficult consultation, talking to a colleague briefly to check management, meditating for a short time on a focus which brings inner peace and preparation, or giving the examination couch a clean round ready for the next person.

The Inner Consultation in this way focuses on astute observation and our internal mechanisms, conflicts, and inner agreements which can enhance or detract from our practice and provides training to GPs to improve performance.

Behaviours that aren't logical

Behaviours that aren't logical may still make sense to the patient. If someone has been subject mainly to illogical or irrational behaviour then they may logically assume this is normal behavior. This is difficult for people to gain insight into, as they would have to experience 'normal' behaviour and then undo their learned responses.

GPs have a scientific background and logical approach; usually it works well. Symptoms and signs don't let us down often. GPs create a logical, hypothetical list of possible diagnoses and then, using deduction, settle on the most likely diagnosis. This in turn leads to rational investigation and management decisions. However, there are a group of patients who attend with more complex dynamics. Sometimes these are insoluble or changing symptoms, or a plethora of conditions in which, as soon as the doctor nears the truth of the condition, they seem to transform and re-present differently. There is also a group of people who, despite the solution to their condition being obvious and achievable, will not follow the medical recommendation but will return to the GP to complain about the problem rather than help themselves. Patients repeatedly acting illogically and/or preventing doctors from solving their problems is frustrating. GPs may even see them deteriorate in health, psychological, or social terms. This is not what we are trained for. When this happens, we hit the buffers and are not sure how to proceed. In short, it is stressful. If the doctor responds by being illogical or irrational back to the patient, it is unprofessional and may lead to complaints. We may flounder in trapped consultations. The GP is, however, blind to the reasoning, emotions and developmental background of the patient and blind to their current social levers. These may have a major bearing on their presentations and actions.

Scenario: A mother who can't reward herself

Mrs X was much doted on by her dad. Every time she did something well at school she was given a present, often a favourite box of chocolates. It is no surprise that she became very obese. Her 10-year-old daughter was unfortunately also obese, leading to reported bullying at school. Despite clear messages about weight loss for the daughter, both mum and daughter remained obese. Mum would reward her daughter with the biggest ice cream she could buy outside school and gave her treats whenever she did well. The treats were so frequent that they were in fact part of her usual diet.

Here the mother knew she was an unhealthy weight but was not able to lose weight for herself. She had never achieved anything for its own sake for herself, only to gain a reward from a loved figure. Success was always accompanied by reward, whether money or food. It was thus unsurprising that she couldn't manage her daughter's weight. Finding the right reward for her health behaviour was a medical enigma as it required a total change in self-view for the mother.

Other people have experienced overbearing parents. The parents have made every important decision for them so that they have difficulty making decisions themselves later in life as adults. This person may want a GP to exhibit authoritarian dogmatism and may struggle to make decisions about their own health care and exert autonomy. Some people can change roles, depending on the circumstances, but some remain rooted in a child learned role. An adult that cannot take responsibility can be very difficult for a GP to handle over time.

Scenario: Alcoholism and misplaced attention

An alcoholic complains of drinking too much, saying she wants to give up but won't. For this patient, the benefit of drinking accrued in the attention, given the next day after a binge, in being told to stop, accompanied by the rigmarole and social dancing about her problem. The misplaced behaviour was not the drinking, it was seeking the attention afterwards. In childhood the only attention given to her had been when being told off and this had been misconstrued as normal, even wanted attention, rather than experiencing parental unconditional love. Sadly, as alcoholism wearies the intellect and creates a premature dementia for many alcoholics, changing this stance becomes more difficult with time. The ability to stand as a mature adult and decide to stop for herself was lost.

Several mature adult patients have described abusive upbringings. In general practice, it is eye-opening to hear how terrible many upbringings are. Some of these survivors reach insight and wisdom, some worry about it and some cannot change their responses and choose adult relationships with the same abuses. What appears to be stupidity or madness, until the GP opens his/her mind to all possibilities, may not be.

Scenario: Wisdom in knowing, but needing confirmation

Mr Y brought his two young daughters to see the GPs frequently with every minor self-healing ailment. These appointments filled up clinics and were frustrating. One day the following was said:

Mr Y: *I bring the kids in a lot, don't I? You always say they are okay and it's just a cold but I don't think I had a good upbringing and I worry that I am not a good father.*

GP: *I don't think you come too often, lots of parents worry about their children. There is nothing in your notes to say you are a poor father and in fact I think you do a very good job. If you want my opinion, that is!*

Mr Y nodded and left. He didn't come as often afterwards.

PERSONAL EXPERIENCE WHICH MAKE PATIENTS AND DOCTORS RISK AVERSE

Despite evidence-based medicine, doctors and patients are influenced by their personal experiences. NHS leaders, wanting us to follow them and their guidelines, call this risk aversion. Others call it learning by anecdote or by experience and feel it is valid. We discuss this more in the ethical section of the book but an example all clinicians will recognise is presented in the following scenario.

Scenario: Knowing the truth but personal experience clouds logic

Mr Y, 22 years old, attends with abdominal pain due to poor diet and stress. He doesn't change behavior and the pain continues. Due to lack of cure, the GP refers him reluctantly to the gastroenterology OPC and he has negative tests. He comes asking for more tests. The GP asks why, when the possibility of any serious illness at his age and with his symptoms is remote. He replies that his granddad had died the year before of bowel cancer and he thinks he has the same symptoms.

GPs recognise patients who have come because their family or friends have frightened them with an anecdote and ended with, 'it could be serious, like cancer', when the symptoms and age group are highly unlikely for the diagnosis. In the same way, a GP who has had an unexpected case, particularly with an adverse outcome, e.g. meningitis, will send patients to secondary care with any signs remotely possible of meningitis until that GP experiences the low incidence of the disease and regains confidence in his/her predictive clinical abilities. Some colleagues may bring patients with quick, easy problems back to see them to avoid seeing acute cases. While this may be a ploy to allow a GP to catch up in time and have an intellectual break, it may be that the GP is anxious and stressed so brings back cases which are unlikely to end in uncertain or adverse outcomes, e.g. BP checks. It is important to recognise this. If a GP is stressed because a case has turned out badly, their colleagues should support them back into full practice.

It is a fact that with time clinicians are likely to become more risk adverse because they have seen more cases. The only GP who will always have good patient outcomes will be the one who sees no patients! GPs should not be measured against one adverse outcome when they have worked to good outcomes for years. It is up to the profession and its employers to support good HCPs. The affected member of the public who has had a poor outcome, perhaps a late diagnosis of cancer, may take issue with the GP. But if this has been unforeseen and the GP has done their best at the time, then the GP should be supported by their practice so that they can manage cases confidently. This requires some planning within the practice and some handholding. It might require a period of joint clinics. Due to time issues GPs don't always offer support to struggling colleagues, who are left to perform at a low level rather than maximizing their skills, and some ultimately retire early.

CRIMINALISATION

Criminalisation of mistakes is rare, but a fear for all GPs. GPs need to be at the top of their game when consulting and use their skills for the good of the patient. They should be self-aware and professional at all times and keep good records. GPs and trainees who write 'no red flags' to indicate that they have asked patients about serious life threatening symptoms should instead make a note of what symptoms were excluded. 'No red flags' is not specific if one is ever asked to defend his/her practice. Red flags refer to symptoms which are discriminators for serious illnesses. If mistakes occur, we should be honest, keep good records, and let our medical defence organisation know.

PATIENTS WHO WON'T LEAVE THE CONSULTATION

Patients who won't leave the consultation are tricky and no one clinician has the answer to this issue. It is difficult not to feel rude, but GPs have a responsibility to all the other patients and to him/herself to keep to time. Those persistent, sitting-in-clinic-for-an-hour individuals are difficult. My best advice is to offer them an end-of-day appointment. Many do respond to doctor comments such as, 'I will have to get on now, I have patients in the waiting room still'.

Continuing consultations are quite different

PATIENT WITH CONTINUING ILLNESS

The patient with a continuing illness hopes that he/she will meet the same clinician throughout their illness. It is easier to talk to the same person without having to back-fill the history, progress and any attendant problems every time the person attends a GP. But in the move to larger general practices and numerous grades of staff able to consult with patients, there is a loss of continuity of care across UK primary care. Many goodwill messages to GPs from patients refer to the continuity and care they have received and appreciated. It is extraordinary how patients rise above their own troubles to thank clinicians for diagnosing their cancers or heart disease because the doctor has kept with them, from initial presentations to secondary care referral and beyond. Unless you are an unusual practice which has plenty of appointment slots, it can be difficult to get an appointment with the same doctor. Patients can gain continuity though if they are brought back by a clinician who thinks it is important that they offer that service.

Scenario: Being sent round the practice

Miss X attended in tears. The GP's previous patient had been in tears so the tissues were on the desk ready. He assumed this was a depressed young patient and asked what was the matter. She replied that she had visited the GP practice three times already. The first time she told the practice nurse about her irregular period problems and the nurse advised Miss X to see a GP. Miss X returned to see a GP, a male partner. The male GP suggested that Miss X required examination and to book in with a female GP. Miss X booked in with a female GP, a locum, who said no time had been allocated for the examination and to rebook. Miss X rebooked and had come into clinic to find a male GP at his desk and burst into tears! My colleague of course acted as her GP and dealt with the patient's concern and of course included the required examination. His comment was that the symptoms could have indicated cancer but in fact the eventual result was no disease. However, it required a GP to do their job.

Consultations which require continuity are often not the most rewarding over the short term, but over decades of practice can be very fulfilling. Treating someone with an asthma attack is immediately fulfilling, while dealing with a patient with difficult lifelong anxiety can be frustrating. There is no detective, no possibility of cure in continuing care of incurable and sometimes untreatable conditions. GPs may need to reevaluate their satisfaction outcomes, moving from a medical model of 'diagnosis-to-cure' to an evaluation of improvements in all areas of the patient's life and supporting them. This is not trendy with NHS leaders as it is difficult to know how much improvement is gained for the NHS's money. Evaluating this in detail might be useful but the thought of another tick box form to prove worth being foisted on GPs does not appeal. In addition, knowing how the patient's year might have turned out without the GP's input is an unknown. In deciding to offer continuity of care ask the following:

- Why am I bringing this patient back?
- What do I hope to achieve?
- Does the patient know why they are returning?
- Do they agree with this plan?
- If I am not here when the patient returns, is the medical record clear about what I intended to do, for the next GP?

Examples of patients requiring continuity of care are those with chronic pain who have tried many medications and arrive hoping for further pain relief. This includes patients with enduring illnesses such as Parkinson's disease or multiple sclerosis, chronic mental health issues, cancer and dementia sufferers. We all want a personal GP even if the issue is considered less important. For example, if we have had an allergic reaction to an antibiotic, we hope that we meet the GP who dealt with that problem and might remember it, because we really can't remember the name of it! If a patient does not need a review then be clear with them; you have gone as far as you can at present and they don't need to routinely return. Some patients find this difficult to accept.

PATIENTS REQUIRING REPEAT MEDICATION REVIEW

Medication reviews require specific GP knowledge on action, side-effects, inter-actions with other medications, benefits, harms, and the patient's views on the medication. Sometimes it seems for GPs that the only important thing we need to know is the cost and if there is a cheaper alternative. Employing pharmacists in practices is common in order to save on drug costs but this may also deskill GPs long-term. It is important that the pharmacist and GP work together as a team.

Recording dates to stop some medications is problematic. For instance, a cardiology opinion over stopping dual antiplatelet therapy (DAPT) such as aspirin and clopidogrel, after a stent has been inserted into a coronary artery for a heart attack, may be personalised. The cardiologist calculates the patient's expected risk of rethrombosis versus bleeding risk and the expected date of cessation is sent in the outpatient clinic (OPC) letter to the GP. This date should be placed on the medication screen. Other medications are recommended for a usual five year course, and again, annotating the drug on the repeat prescription screen with a cessation date, when the GP has long forgotten why it was started, is important.

Patients may not take all their medications. A patient with moderately severe chronic obstructive pulmonary disease (COPD) admitted that he had stopped all his inhalers, except his salbutamol inhaler, because they didn't seem to help. He might be right of course, so this requires discussion. The discussion arose because the GP noted that the last inhaler prescription printout was dated four months ago, rather than one month ago. The patient had not brought the topic up despite attending with a cough, but it was clear from the medication records. Some patients take their medications just before their HCP check-up appointment and this may cause problems in blood test interpretations, as well as not offering disease control. For example, a patient should be taking levothy-roxine tablets regularly for hypothyroidism but in fact only took them for the week before the recommended thyroid function blood test. They had not been taken for weeks before then. This resulted in a normal levothyroxine level but a raised thyroid-stimulating hormone level. Interpreting this patient as requir-ing more levothyroxine would be erroneous; in this case it was lack of adher-ence. Another patient admitted to taking his atorvastatin for only one month before his annual check-up blood test so that he didn't upset his GP. He enjoyed eating a high-fat diet and didn't take his atorvastatin at other times. He felt the GP did a good job for him but he wanted to choose which bit of that good job he followed. However, he didn't want to upset his GP and not feel able to see him if needed. Another patient disclosed that he sold his sildenafil (Viagra) down the pub!

A carer told her GP on a home visit that she was reluctant to stop her husband's Alzheimer's medication even though she felt it was ineffective for him. This was because if the medication was stopped, the dementia nurse would no longer visit. The visits of the specialist dementia nurse were linked in this particular service to patients on dementia medications. The medication, being sadly ineffective, was stopped. When the dementia sufferer reached end of life, the carer phoned the secondary care help numbers, including the dementia nurse number given to her, and was told that her husband had been discharged from care and none was forthcoming. Had she continued with the medication for her husband, the nurse would have been available. Patient decisions can be complex and unforeseen by medical teams.

Other people may forget to take their medications. Some may not understand how their medications work and so stop it, thinking they have completed a course. Some people may never have agreed to take it. Forgetful patients may need medication dispensed in weekly monitored dosage systems (MDS) with the days and time clearly marked. During home visits there is an opportunity to count tablets in bottles if patients are not improving. Sometimes they have not taken the tablets despite professing to adhere to treatment. GP records show when the patient has requested prescriptions and GPs can include a minimum interval before the patient can get the next prescription. This is helpful in preventing medication overuse.

There are some medications (referred to as red drugs) which are only prescribed in secondary care. GPs are deskilled in these medications and they may be missing from the repeat prescription screen. Interactions may then be missed when the GP prescribes for the patient. Red drugs should be included on the repeat prescription chart. Whilst medications which GPs are prescribing repeatedly should be added to the repeat prescription screen, so should regular over-the-counter (OTC) medications. These can be marked as OTC, and put as not for printing, not for dispensing, with no volume of prescription and with no repeat issues. However, it does then provide a full visible record of the patient's medications. Commonly bought OTC medications are vitamins, antihistamines, paracetamol and aspirin. Also patients are more commonly buying prescription medications online.

SEXUAL, OBSTETRIC AND GYNAECOLOGICAL HISTORIES

Consultations in sexual (male and female), gynaecological, and obstetric health are different to the routine medical consultations we learn. Asking sexually explicit questions of a man or woman is a specific skill set. In asking these questions doctors must be certain they are not being misinterpreted by the patient and attract complaints of sexual misbehaviour. This is particularly true for male doctors with female patients, but not exclusively. When being asked about periods, sex, contraception, vaginal discharge, and risks of STIs patients are understandably embarrassed and may be shocked. GPs may need to ask about possible abuse. In asking personal questions GPs should warn the patient using a general statement so that they are mentally prepared. Make questions and statements impersonal and professional to ensure the patient realises the questioning is relevant to their presentation.

Scenario: Vaginal discharge

Miss X: I have come over a smelly discharge that I've got down below.

GP: You mean a vaginal discharge? How long have you had this?

Miss X: Two weeks.

GP: Can you tell me anything else about it?

Miss X: Not really.

GP: I am going to ask you some personal questions now which I need to know about if that's okay? Firstly, are your periods normal?

Miss X: Yes.

GP: When was your last period? Are they regular, or do you have bleeding in between?

Miss X: Two weeks ago, and yes, they are monthly.

GP: Is there any chance you could be pregnant?

Miss X: None

GP: Why is that?

Miss X: I don't have a boyfriend.

GP: Okay, so you are not having sex then? So, you are not worried about sexually transmitted infections?

Miss X: No, it's just I have this smell.

GP: Okay, well I have to ask. Lastly, are you on any contraception at present then?

A bit more questioning and this patient sounded like she had bacterial vaginosis. The discharge was offensive and she was up to date with cervical cytology screening. The GP treated her with metronidazole as the smell of organic acids being metabolized was diagnostic of an anaerobic organism, consistent with gardnerella in bacterial vaginosis. If the patient returned, due to failure to cure, she understood she would require examination and swabs.

Obstetric histories require personal questioning about previous miscarriages, contraception and births including baby gestation at birth, mode of delivery and past breast feeding. Again, the GP should introduce a professional statement such as, 'I am now going to ask you some personal questions which are relevant'.

MENTAL HEALTH HISTORIES

Despite being trained in mental health histories, it is the intense personal intrusion which can delay or prevent doctors asking relevant questions. In practice, patients are often pleased to talk about their distressing symptoms. Patients who appear depressed should be sensitively asked about their home circumstances, who is home, and how useful is their presence in helping them day by day. There may be concerns about whether the depressed person is getting the children up for school, giving them breakfast, etc. But there are also depressed people who the GP finds have realised the problems and have moved mum into the house to help them!

Questions should step up, asking:

- Is he/she weepy?
- Do he/she think they are depressed?
- How depressed is he/she?
- Has he/she become morbid?
- Has he/she thought about harming themselves or tried to do this?

Ask for more details if people answer in the affirmative. There are useful score charts for depression but they can also become a tick box substitute for listening and consulting well. When asked about suicide one patient surprisingly pulled a suicide note out of his shirt pocket. Another patient placed his shopping bag on the desk and took out several packets of paracetamol with which he had intended to kill himself. When asked why he had shown the tablets to the GP he said he had come to say goodbye. The GP then asked to look in his bag and found more packets of paracetamol and arranged his admission to the mental health team. Again, questions should be ring-fenced by warning patients that questions are personal but relevant. Patients with psychosis can have very specific thought disorders and asking patients whether they have unusual thoughts, what they are, and whether they have visual or auditory hallucinations takes time and skill. Many upset people report thinking 'abnormal thoughts' and being oversensitive, but not all are psychotic. Cultural backgrounds may influence patient's experiences.

Delusions are strongly held abnormal convictions. For example, a patient may have grandiose delusions, when someone is convinced they are God or a monarch. Or conversely, delusions of poverty in which, despite all evidence, they believe they have no money at all. Paranoid delusions might refer to a belief that 'someone is out to get them', e.g. a terrorist group or special police force. On visiting a patient and uncovering a psychosis a GP was told he was 'evil and had come to get the patient', The consultation was becoming threatening so the GP left quickly, returning with the police and psychiatric team to section him.

In thought disorder, some people cannot think logically so it is difficult to follow their train of thought or speech. People may feel that their thoughts are inserted by someone else. Thoughts may be controlled by others, sometimes by waves from the radio, laptop, TV or mobile phone. Thoughts may appear to be taken away from them by others.

Auditory hallucinations, i.e. hearing voices so realistic that they appear to be real, can be very intrusive and unsettling. Patients may visibly turn round repeatedly, responding to the voice. These voices vary but may give the person unpleasant messages about themselves or others, and may issue commands to injure others.

Visual hallucinations are seeing things which just aren't there, people or animals. They can occur in dementia, delirium, alcoholism, including delirium tremens and psychosis.

Even when stable some people with psychosis continue to experience some mental abnormalities but at a lesser intensity and frequency. They may recognise these experiences as abnormal and continue to function as themselves. This must be difficult to do.

In mental health histories we develop skills in finding these abnormalities. We need to be firm and professional in asking questions over alcohol and drug misuse. Patients should be asked how they are affected by their symptoms and what they would like to happen to help them. It may be that the GP needs to use a section of the Mental Health Act (MHA) but often people are willing to be helped by voluntary admission and assessment. Patients with dementia need to be heard, and so does the carer. As the population ages, GPs rely heavily on carers, who are themselves often elderly, to maintain their loved ones with dementia at home. These consultations, as with parents and young children, require a three-way discussion and management plan.

BREAKING BAD NEWS

This phrase, 'breaking bad news', is often reserved for cancer diagnoses but can refer to any bad news. It is important to understand what the patient is thinking and to offer a return appointment to discuss the questions the 'breaking bad news' consultation has engendered. These questions won't be present immediately – people have to think through the consequences of bad news. When someone is told they have cancer they may need silence to take the news in. Their next question is often:

What can you do about it? What is the plan? How bad is it? Doctors should pre-empt this when breaking bad news, but do not lose sight of the patient's symptoms either. The patient may be told for instance that they have pancreatic cancer but their goal, at that moment, may be to stop being repeatedly sick and nauseated.

The consultation should not be interrupted, which is true of all consultations, but particularly one where people are having to think through bad news. GPs should be prepared for anger and upset. This may be directed at them, but we advise not to automatically use this as a reason not to offer continuity. Patients and their families are grateful that GPs stick with them and do their best for them. Patients usually want to be offered hope. This is a realistic hope within the limits of their condition, and to be told about problems clearly in a way they understand. Giving written information, referral to cancer websites, and copies of GP or hospital letters may be helpful.

Breaking bad news is not always about cancer. Telling a parent her child has T1IDD, that a son has schizophrenia, or a newly retired man has COPD, or CHD, or multiple sclerosis, etc. is also breaking bad news. As doctors we can be insensitive to the labels we place on patients and how they receive the messages we give. We may not understand the significance of a non-cancer diagnosis in someone's life. GPs may over-emphasise the positive aspects of a diagnosis and therapy, as this fulfils our roles as doctors. We may not appreciate the full implications and ideas that patients and family members may have about a condition.

In delivering a serious adverse diagnosis like cancer, there are sometimes two scenarios.

One relates to patients who have no idea they have cancer and the other to patients who attend because they are concerned about cancer, e.g. they have a breast lump.

In the first situation the GP needs to suggest the possibility first, with further discussion after confirmatory tests. This can be a problem if the patient is being referred on a cancer 2 week wait (2WW) form, so that the patient is seen in the cancer clinic within two weeks. In this circumstance, the GP may state on the form that the patient is not aware of the likely diagnosis and why. The form makes it clear that GPs should let patients know they are referred on a 2WW form and, whenever possible, this should happen. Occasionally there are a few patients for whom at that moment it is a step too far.

Scenario: Patient does not suspect colorectal cancer

Before Mr Y, 70 years old, entered his clinic the GP noticed on the patient's history screen that his last attendance six weeks before had been with a few days of diarrhoea and a colleague had diagnosed gastroenteritis. Mr Y was generally fit with no medications or chronic illnesses.

Mr Y: I've got diarrhoea and I had it a few weeks ago. It went with loperamide. Can I have some more?

This patient was blind to the idea of a cancer but on abdominal examination the GP found a right iliac fossa mass and Mr Y looked anaemic. When the GP discussed excluding serious causes of repeated diarrhoea, and pointed out the finding of an abdominal lump, Mr Y stated that he was certain it was food poisoning. Indeed, he had cooked some liver the night before but thought it was 'off' as his dog hadn't eaten any!

This was of course a classic caecal colonic cancer. Mr Y had bloods taken and a 2WW colorectal referral made, but the form was clearly marked that he didn't think he had a cancer. He did very well with treatment.

Scenario: Patient does not suspect incurable advanced lung cancer

Mr Y is 85 years old and fit but attends the GP with recent onset numerous hard nodules appearing under the skin. To the GP this was certainly secondary lung cancer in the skin and chest examination confirmed this. The patient had come asking what the skin lumps were but the GP decided it was unkind to tell him at that moment, as he was not expecting an advanced terminal cancer diagnosis. The GP introduced the idea that it could be due to serious illness and that cancer could be a cause. An urgent chest X-ray (CXR) and 2WW referral was made with a GP follow up appointment for two weeks later. However, the diagnosis, though certain, was not forced upon Mr Y at that first consultation.

In primary care GPs stating a cancer diagnosis and suggesting a cancer diagnosis are very different consultations. In the above scenario, Mr Y needed to see a specialist but there is unlikely to be any active treatment possible. The patient's mindset was so far removed from death and cancer that it would have been cruel to force the conversation at that point. Offering a return appointment to go through the diagnosis and care is of course needed.

Scenario: Patient does not suspect gastric cancer on tests
Mrs X, 60 years old, attended hospital for investigations and had a biopsy. She attends a GP for the result. The GP doesn't know her and hasn't got the result but, being helpful, finds the result, which is one of cancer. The GP is personally shocked at the news and is now faced with telling the patient, who has attended alone, that she has cancer but is unable to provide a follow-on plan. The patient became angry and upset. The GP was also upset.

For patients who think they have cancer, the consultation is very different. The discussion can be more frank. Patients appreciate clear management and follow up plans. The role of the GP is often to optimize the patient's mental and physical health so that they can cope best with cancer therapy and function to the best of their abilities. In many 'breaking bad news' consultations patients have already weighed their symptoms and decided that they need the GP to rule out cancer, or that they are likely to have cancer. Being clear and open with patients about investigations and their likelihood of cancer is important. GPs will mainly know which patients have definitely got cancer and which are unlikely to have it based on symptoms and signs. A patient with a hard, irregular, fixed mass is likely to have a cancer. A patient with symptoms which can be attributable to many benign conditions and with no abnormal signs is unlikely to have cancer. In these consultations patients appreciate the opportunity to discuss their concerns and fears. They appreciate that the doctor is trying to ensure they do not have a serious disease and they may want to decide how much investigation is appropriate.

Unfortunately, not all cancers are cured and the laws and regulations section discusses regulatory frameworks which help in advanced care planning and end of life care which can be introduced into the consultation. All these may be pertinent to cancer consultations if there is a terminal prognosis.

Giving away consultations and curriculum

GPs are unique in 'seeing everything' related to health care in its widest possible sense and sticking with families and individuals for the long term. This is not a target-driven, ego-led career. It is a career which has immense long-term positive health outcomes for people. This can be very difficult to measure. General practice has become less popular as a career and there is an urgent need to rediscover and redefine GP consultations and the GP curriculum. The RCGP has a good GP curriculum but it is very wide and does not fully represent the activities of today's GPs.

GPs should define their tasks, publicise them to patients, to secondary care, and to other HCPs, and be widely supported by politicians and organisations who inspect, inform and maintain the system. GPs, as professionals, need to decide which consultations they want to delegate, why, and how this will affect their jobs and patient care. In the past this has happened without looking carefully at the pros and cons of giving aspects of medicine away to others and making definite choices within the profession. An obvious example of giving away skills is in midwifery. GPs used to enjoy antenatal clinics and helping midwives at straightforward births; this made a change from illness and death and meant that they knew young mothers and family circumstances. Midwifery has taken over antenatal and intrapartum care of patients completely. Or has it? Do patients who are pregnant still come to GPs? Do GPs feel confident treating them? Pregnant women do still come to GPs and GPs are deskilled in managing their problems and so are more likely to make mistakes and offer suboptimal care. Perhaps midwives should see all pregnant women, at all times? Or should there be an acknowledgement that GPs require revision in obstetrics over their careers, as they will have low obstetric problem consultation rates and will not be highly skilled when consulted? There are a number of responses to this problem, but for now it is enough to ask the questions of the reader:

What exactly do GPs do and not do for a living?

How can they best maintain skills in all they do?

A second example is in end of life care. At one time this was almost entirely delivered by GPs with district nurse help and then changed to be delivered mainly by district nurses and has recently changed to a balanced, shared care with GPs. It is unfortunate that district nurses have often been moved out of GP premises in reorganisations, so there is less opportunity to develop long-term team-working. A GP told a patient that district nurses no longer 'do personal care'. District nurses may have a different opinion but this illustrates the difficulties of not working closely!

Patients are now triaged by so many other HCPs doing parts of a GP's job that many GPs are confused and uncertain about which person does what and how much responsibility they can take upon themselves if working within general practice.

If GPs give their 'easy' consultations and skills away, what are they left with?

GPs now lack 'easy' skills in ear syringing, phlebotomy, suturing, glues, dressings, SC and intramuscular (IM) injections, and cervical cytology (smears). Patients attending for these are referred to other HCPs. Management of algorithmic care, e.g. patients with eczema, psoriasis, asthma, COPD, hypertension and diabetes are often delegated to other HCPs. As these conditions and skills are taken over, not shared, GPs become deskilled and younger doctors entering primary care do not gain experience of responses to eczema therapy, etc. Secondary care, perhaps failing to trust GPs, send specialised hospital nurses out into the community to manage diabetics, heart failure, and COPD patients.

GPs are generally left with untreatable, chronic, less rewarding complaints such as 'hypertension cases which won't reach target', chronic depression, and anxiety states. There are many intellectual sequelae to this for the profession. Some medical students have complained that this is the main content of their experience when sitting with GPs as part of undergraduate education. The conundrum is that GPs actually see and manage lots of illness and are overworked, and yet lots of GP functions are now delegated. An investigation into the core skills of GPs and those of their teams might provide direction and clarity for the profession.

Keeping GP skills up to date over a 35-year career, when medicine changes quite quickly, and defining how GPs work with other HCPs would be helpful. Many patients attending primary care recover whoever sees them and this confounds organisers when deciding how to manage primary care. Lastly, the reader will realise that a 10-minute consultation is often inappropriate to offer high value primary care consultations.

3

Knowledge and evidence

'*The manager does things right, the leader does the right thing*'.

Warren Dennis, 1925–2014, American author and academic

General practitioners (GPs) are inundated with guidance and this section explores guidelines, including why and how we do or do not use guidance as GPs, especially within the consultation. It also offers a number of useful resources, some of which may be helpful to have on the desktop in clinics. I discuss critical analysis of information, using QRISK2 as an example and how it may relate to patients and I discuss problems which occur with information over time, e.g. individual experiences versus evidence and common prescribing issues.

Although most GPs are not statistical experts some statistical terms are discussed with examples of how interpretation of data can be problematic, e.g. altering according to prevalence or the statistic used.

This section is not a clinical or statistical textbook. As always there are useful resources to help GPs look into interesting areas in more depth.

Size of information

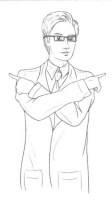

That's good guidance!

KNOWING THAT WE CAN'T KNOW

GPs require accurate, up-to-date knowledge in order to present accurate information to their patients and help them make best decisions about their care. As students, we are taught basic anatomy and physiology and onto this we scaffold our learning of body systems, diseases, medications, etc. Some facts, like the usual route of the sciatic nerve, are unchanging. However, many facts change over time and, over the last 15 years, medicine has entered an exciting era of fast-moving molecular biology. This has transformed our understanding of inflammation and cancer with insights into molecular mechanisms interacting between immunology, inflammation and tumours. Using this information brilliant researchers have developed many new medications to alleviate inflammatory disorders, like rheumatoid arthritis, and to destroy cancer cells. These targeted therapies include tyrosine kinase inhibitors and the biologics like monoclonal antibodies. The more that is understood and learned over time, the more we marvel at the intricate mechanisms balancing health within our bodies and the positive progress in conditions which were previously difficult to improve. GPs cannot prove that everything they are taught is correct; as life-long learners we rely and believe expert curriculums, books, journals, online sites, expert organisations, study days and drug representatives. There is, therefore, a degree of trust and maybe 'magic' involved.

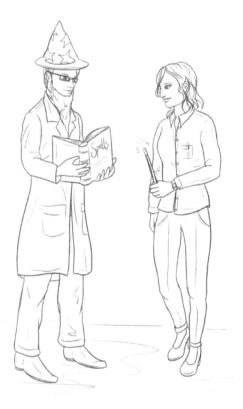

Magic and medicine

Accepting facts: Insulin and pioglitazone

In 1921 Banting and Best discovered that injecting insulin derived from a dog pancreas into dogs lowered their blood sugar. From this they developed insulin, a life-saving therapy for type 1 diabetics. This is accepted as fact and conforms with observed practice. About 10 years ago a drug for T2DM appeared, called pioglitazone. It is one of a group of medications called glitazones or thiazolidinediones. Pioglitazone acts through peroxisome proliferator-activated receptors (PPARs).

Peroxisomes are small organelles in cells which are very active and have many functions related to lipid metabolism. The mechanism of action of pioglitazone has been described as follows:

Pioglitazone improves glycaemic control in people with type 2 diabetes by improving insulin sensitivity through its action at PPARγ1 and PPARγ2, and affects lipid metabolism through action at PPAR alpha. The results of these interactions include: increases in glucose transporters 1 and 4, lowered free fatty acids, enhanced insulin signalling, reduced tumour necrosis factor alpha (TNFα), and remodelling of adipose tissue. Together, these can increase glucose uptake and utilisation in the peripheral organs and decrease gluconeogenesis in the liver, thereby reducing insulin resistance.*

PPAR, peroxisomes, glucose transporter 1 and 4, insulin signalling and even TNFα are new concepts for most GPs and if we don't understand them, the information must be accepted at face value.

There is no uniform mechanism for knowledge updates. There are annual appraisals in which to display knowledge and skills which have been revised or newly learned but they do not cover the full GP knowledge base and changes. A GP running family planning services in their practice will keep up to date in family planning. However, if a patient with a urinary tract infection, who is also diabetic, wants to discuss rising blood sugars, that GP may feel uncomfortable about the extent of their knowledge and may not be very familiar with the latest diabetic medications. Patients attend primary care with anything and everything; this means generalist knowledge is very important and gaps can cause uncertainty and stress for GPs. Also lack of detailed knowledge in this multitude of areas inhibits critical review of guidelines, evidence and questioning of information by jobbing GPs. It can be difficult to know which guidance to take on and which to reject as not useful or relevant. In the last 10 years, the introduction of 12-hour ambulatory BP monitoring (ABPM) for diagnosis of hypertension and exclusion of white coat hypertension, use of CA125 for the early detection of ovarian cancer and the use of C-reactive protein (CRP) to prove or disprove the likelihood of bacterial chest infections and improve the use of antibiotics have been a few of the useful changes in clinical practice. Interestingly, many are advances in primary care investigations,

---

* Smith U. Pioglitazone: mechanism of action. *Int J Clin Pract Suppl.* 2001 September;**121**:13–18.

enhancing clinical decision making at times of uncertainty and shortening the diagnostic route, e.g. to hypertension. Computers arrived in the late 1980s, the world wide web in the early 1990s, and Google in the late 1990s. A search at our university library online in 2017 for 'primary prevention in hypertension' reveals 794 search results when searching up to 1990, 12,423 up to 2010 and 21,129 when searching up to 2017. A search on 'hypertension' reveals 1,796,080 results in 2017. Being able to share and engage with knowledge online leads to much more knowledge being available worldwide. Yet this makes it more difficult for GPs to know what is worthwhile reading and what is not. Usually our decisions are based on what interests us and seems relevant.

SELECTING INFORMATION

GPs select the sources of information that they find easiest to assimilate and use in their daily work.

This may include seeing pharmaceutical representatives (drug reps) and many updated sessions are sponsored by drug companies providing meals and financial help, providing the drug rep has a short platform to talk to their medical audience. This happens at national and practice levels and GPs may be unduly influenced by drug reps. Most doctors say that they are not influenced, but one needs to be wary of intellectual conceit. Drug reps would not exist if they were not effective communicators of their company's products.

Many agencies provide clinical knowledge updates, e.g. RCGP knowledge updates, GP journals, update courses (online and in person), and clinical guidelines, of which the major resource is the National Institute for Health and Care Excellence (NICE). These and others provide clinical guidance.

Points to consider in deciding what to read are as follows:

- Is this guidance from a source I respect?
- Is this guidance relevant to my clinical practice and development?
- Is this guidance relevant to my practice population?
- Am I motivated to read it? Am I open to confirming my practice as good or changing my practice if there is new advice?
- Is it easy to access? Is it an easy read? Is it short?
- Is it easy to fit into usual primary care practice?

We may read a round-up journal or we may access NICE, Scottish Intercollegiate Guideline Network (SIGN), or other major guideline producers. There are three levels of information:

1. Those we use routinely in clinic
2. Those we want immediate access to but don't use regularly
3. Those we want to be able to access for learning but do not usually access in a clinic slot

Below are some useful links which GPs may put on their desktop for use in clinic:

1. NHS Evidence at https://www.evidence.nhs.uk/. This site acts as a search engine to lead to other sites like NICE or BNF. We can access the BNF separately at https://www.medicinescomplete.com/mc/bnf/64 and selecting the BNF from the drop down menu.

2. Our local Primary Care Antibiotic Formulary is derived from Public Health England's (PHE) annual national guidance *Managing Common Infections in Primary Care* and altered for local resistance and sensitivities: https://www.gov.uk/government/uploads/system/uploads/attachment_data/file/586767/managing_common_infections_summary.pdf.

3. Online calculator for patients who bring in lists of readings from home blood pressure monitoring (HBPM) as their method of BP assessment. Also, a metric-imperial converter for patients jumping on your metric scales who then ask what it means in stones and pounds.

Other favourites which provide quick access to information and may be useful within the consultation:

4. Family Planning Association (FPA) Leaflets online at http://www.fpa.org.uk/resources/leaflet-and-booklet-downloads. Instead of having to search the practice or find that we have run out of FPA leaflets using this resource, GPs and patients can check the information together on the desktop and so also train the patient to use the leaflet themselves online before contacting the surgery for advice.

5. a. Vaccination schedule (2017) at https://www.gov.uk/government/uploads/system/uploads/attachment_data/file/633693/Complete_imm_schedule_2017.pdf
   and
   b. The Green Book Immunisation against infectious disease by PHE for vaccination queries at https://www.gov.uk/government/collections/immunisation-against-infectious-disease-the-green-book.

6. The UK Medical Eligibility Criteria for Contraceptive Use (UKMEC) 2016 file from the Faculty of Sexual Reproductive Health Care (FRHC) at https://www.fsrh.org/standards-and-guidance/.
   This can be helpful to explore relative risks in contraceptive prescribing.

7. GP COG, general practitioner assessment of cognition at http://gpcog.com.au/ is a favourite because of its speed. It takes a few minutes to assess a patient's cognition and decide whether it might be impaired using the 'begin test' button with the patient before you on the home page.

8. HbA1c converter is available as some longstanding diabetics still struggle with the 'new' units.

9. The Notifications of Infectious Diseases at PHE has a list of notifiable diseases and a click onto the form to fill in to notify a disease at: https://www.gov.uk/government/collections/notifications-of-infectious-diseases-noids.

10. Useful resources for patients are
    a. Patient information at http://patient.info/ which also has a professional link.

    b. The British Hypertension Society has an online home BP diary from
       http://www.bhsoc.org/files/8514/1088/8028/Home_blood_pressure
       _diary.pdf for patients to complete.
    c. There is a peak flow diary for printout for patients to complete at http://
       patient.info/health/asthma-peak-flow-diary.

11. Useful algorithms from NICE guidelines or local CCG clinical governance
    groups. Favourites are on polymyalgia rheumatic (PMR) and headache
    management but GPs will collect their own, dictated by practice preva-
    lence, constancy of guidance over years, and inner knowledge. You may
    have leaflets you have written yourself and use in clinic to drop onto your
    desktop for ease of use. In other sections of this book are links to the Driver
    and Vehicle Licensing Authority (DVLA) fitness to drive information and
    palliative care advice and treatment. Useful resources are linked to sections
    and placed underneath.

If a GP has a specific interest in a topic he/she may want to access the original
trials and apply critical analytical skills outside of the clinic situation. There are
many guidance bodies and update journals which GPs can access in electrons
or paper. The problem isn't always finding resources; it's knowing which ones to
unsubscribe from.

There are two aspects to incorporating information from new guidelines into
clinical practice:

Step 1: Committing to the guideline with a professional decision to change
       practice
Step 2: Detailed, easy to access, and implemented primary care guidelines for
       change or confirmation of management, i.e. the usability of guidance.

Step 1: Committing to a guideline

Personal and institutional bias may affect how we view guidance.

There are sources of bias, even before we approach the patient with our
guidance. The first is the duty of care taken by authorities, whether it is the
government wanting to promote a particular health agenda or pharmaceutical companies wanting to promote positive trial findings to sell medications,
omitting other trials or not performing them in the first place. An organisation, AllTrials at http://alltrials.net, calls for and encourages the registration
of all data, including unpublished clinical trials, to improve total knowledge
and to try to prevent bias. Journals and online medical sites, some more
explicitly drug company sponsored than others, may promote their spon-
sors, offering advertisements of one drug rather than another, whilst offering
knowledge updates. It is possible that people sitting on guideline committees have a biased view or a definite conflict of interest due to pharmaceutical

sponsorship in research, or have had free trips as speakers and free lunches, or perhaps have made friends with the drug company representatives. There is a site, Who pays this doctor? at http://www.whopaysthisdoctor.org/, on which any of us can register our conflicts of interest; but our organisations may also have a database.

It may be the reader, however, who has bias. They may be influenced by drug company representatives or have cultural or clinical bias from their own illness experience.

I have heard students and doctors stating that they would want an antibiotic for a cough because they had previously developed pneumonia and it is 'wrong' to withhold antibiotic prescriptions. This is despite a lack of evidence-based clinical trial data to show any benefit of taking antibiotics for a simple cough. I have heard senior medical students say, 'Get a good lawyer' or 'Go to Spain to stock up!', which is amusing but illustrates the depth of belief that doctors and trainees can hold on to, despite evidence to the contrary.

Once we have decided that we trust the guideline and will read it with an open mind, then we commit to reading it and potentially applying it to our patients and our own practices.

Step 2: Usability of guidance

First, guidance should be easily accessible. NICE and other guideline authorities have made steps to improve usability. Map of Medicine and NICE have illness journey maps that can be clicked through but can sometimes be unwieldy. NICE has a 'tools and resources' section which may include an e-learning module, a useful 'do not do' quick read and a quick link to access algorithms. I recommend the 'do not do' sections as a quick win for practice improvement. Access it at https://www.nice.org.uk/savingsandproductivity/collection?page=1&pagesize =2000&type=do%20not%20do.

Searching for information requires patience and time, with a number of computer clicks required to drill down to advice. If after a few clicks we are advised to click yet again to link to another guidance we may disinvest, log out and leave the guideline unused. GPs want guidelines to serve our patient populations yet in trial work, patients with multiple complex interacting problems and medications are usually excluded. This means that problems due to the index drug can be more obvious. However, once a drug is prescribed to cohorts of complex patients on other medications, adverse reactions and side-effects may become more obvious. The MHRA regularly updates GPs by email, if subscribed, to serious drug interactions but this still leaves us wondering whether the evidence fits our patient. There has been a move nationally to respecting that not all guidance fits all patients, and giving GPs and other guideline users the opportunity to offer personalised medicine and personalised targets for their patients. These should be decided in conjunction with the patient, taking all information and views into account. It is a way of moving a study population finding into a real-world unique patient situation.

Scenario: HbA1c targets in T2DM

Mrs X, 72 years old, has had T2DM for 20 years and has always taken metformin 500 mg tds and gliclazide 80 mg od. She has never had hypoglycaemic attacks and her diabetes HbA1c has been running at 52 mmol/mol. However, as she has aged, her kidney function has started to decline and is now 45 mls/min. Her diabetic lead practice nurse and GP in the practice recommend reducing her metformin and this leads the GP to wonder whether her HbA1c will rise and what she should then do about this.

NICE recommends in 2017 that HbA1c control is as near to non-diabetic levels as possible and recommends a target HbA1c 48 mmol/mol (6.5%).

NICE also recommends that if HbA1c is 58 mmol/mol (7.5%) or higher on one drug, then medication should be increased to reach a reduced HbA1c of 53 mmol/mol (7%).

Also, NICE states, 'Consider relaxing the target HbA1c on a case-by-case basis, with particular consideration for people who are older or frail, for adults with type 2 diabetes' and then goes on to give further advice. This direction respects problems GPs and their teams have in striving for specific targets. Whilst Mrs X may reach her targets, it allows a leeway in patients who have complex needs and is very welcome.

USING FIGURES OF BENEFIT AND RISK OF HARM IN GENERAL PRACTICE

It would be very helpful if ballpark numbers for benefits and harms were included in all guidelines. However, authorities are wary of providing ballpark numbers that may need to be changed with the next published study. It still does not guarantee the clinician or the patient that the disease or the treatment benefit or harm will or will not occur for that individual. Offering an approximation of effect and harm does however improve decision making and knowledge for GPs, and is essential for good shared decision making with patients.

Scenario: Risks of diarrhoea on amoxicillin

Miss X is 25 years old and wants amoxicillin for her chest infection. She has had it before and it worked well for her. On examination, she has a clear chest and slight cough during the consultation. The GP says that the infection is going due to her own immune system activity and that there is no requirement for an antibiotic. Mrs X is disappointed and says, 'They don't have side-effects and they work for me!' The GP asks her to return if she is not recovered in a week but afterwards wonders what the side-effects of amoxicillin are in numbers.

The GP later looks up the MHRA Medicines Information: product details online at http://www.mhra.gov.uk/spc-pil/index.htm and reaches the alphabetical index. On inputting amoxicillin, the patient information leaflet (PIL) comes up and the summary of product characteristics (SPC). Using the reference ranges, e.g. common is between 1 in 10 to 1 in 100, she notes that diarrhoea is a common side-effect but that vomiting is uncommon, occurring in 1 in 100 to 1 in 1,000 users.

Scenario: Starting clindamycin

Mrs X attends the GP to start clindamycin as requested by the orthopaedic special-ist outpatient clinic (OPC) letter. It requests the GP to 'start at a low dose and check the liver enzymes periodically'.

The GP wonders what 'low dose' means and what 'periodically' means.

Using a drug which we are not familiar with is a possible recipe for disaster and asking secondary care colleagues to send detailed management plans to GPs is important. The MHRA Medicines Information site, however, provides a lot of information and covers interactions with other medications.

Using numbers needed to treat (NNT) and numbers needed to harm (NNH) in assessing benefits and harms of medications can be very helpful. For instance, in suggesting the use of aspirin to prevent heart disease in healthy populations, ballpark figures are: 99.94% saw no benefit and 0.03% were harmed by developing a major bleeding event. This figure is accessed at THE NNT online at http://www.thennt.com/. Again, we are trusting the information on the site but it is quick to access, provides information in different formats and does not expect GPs to be statisticians.

Some of the National Screening Committee (NSC) leaflets sent to patients are excellent examples of offering balanced information as it is known now. Usually statistics are presented as numbers of people benefitting; '*1 in 35 people will get*'... for example. I am not aware of a better set of leaflets. The site also has a timeline listing the national screening programme. There have been a number of additions to neonatal screening tests over recent years. The site is '*Population screening programmes: leaflets and how to order them*' at: https://www.gov.uk/government/collections/population-screening-programmes-leaflets-and-how-to-order-them#professional-information-leaflets.

Scenario: Screening for aortic aneurysm

Mr X is 65 years old and receives a leaflet inviting him for aortic aneurysm screening by ultrasound scan. The leaflet describes the screening programme and presents ballpark figures of 'around 1 in 70 men who are screened have an aortic aneurysm.'

Also, 'about 1 in 1,000 men who are screened have a large aneurysm'.

The leaflet describes hazards as, 'However, around 54 out of every 10,000 men screened will eventually have surgery to repair an aneurysm. On average, one of these 54 men will not survive the operation but their aneurysm may never have burst if left untreated. Screening does not completely remove the risk of an aneurysm bursting but it is the best method of protection against this condition'.

In this scenario, Mr X is told he has a small aneurysm and is given infor-mation and the NSC leaflet on 'small aneurysms' which states that '*Around 1 in*

80 men who are screened have a small AAA'. The leaflet also gives advice on family members, driving and health insurance and is very comprehensive.

Outcomes of procedures are not always readily available but for years patients have been asked by questionnaire how they have felt and functioned after hip and knee replacements, varicose vein and groin hernia surgery. These are known as Patient Recorded Outcome Measures (PROMs) and there are three measures used per procedure. NHS Digital has these recorded quarterly and annually at: http://content.digital.nhs.uk/proms and they can be very useful to provide approximate figures of benefit for these procedures, all of which are usually elective and not mandatory for patients, to aid discussion.

RISK SCORES

One of the ways figures are used to predict a patient's risk of disease or a specific condition is by using risk calculators. These have mushroomed over the last few years and can be both an annoying substitute for thinking and a boon for offering figures for benefits and harms for specific conditions. We will look at a tool that GPs use to predict the patient's risk of CVD: QRISK2, a risk stratification tool based upon a UK population.

There is no 'no risk' in health. An example is the controversy within general practice recently around 'prediabetes'. GPs and their patients want to know whether they are diabetic or not. If they are not diabetic they do not expect the adverse consequences, medically or socially, of being a diabetic. However, the cut-off HbA1c or blood glucose for diagnosing T2DM is just an arbitrary cut-off, and the threshold should be whether the risk is considered high or low by the patient. Using a lower pre-risk concept has led to an escalator image of increasing risk of diabetes with rising HbA1c. Therefore, there are people with 'high-normal' HbA1c, who might consider themselves prediabetic. The question for doctors, patients, national groups and governments is: what are the sequelae of labelling more people with a health problem in terms of harms and benefits?

How do we decide a cut-off point at which the remaining risk of harm is acceptable to people and society?

Choose Wisely and the RCGP over-diagnosis group have formed in the last few years, largely in response to concerns about over-diagnosis, over-investigation and over-treatments, and they encourage debate and publicity about best practice.

Traditionally doctors have taken a detailed history and examination and used these to decide how at risk someone is of an illness, or future illness. Risk tool makers synthesise the most common and important of these risk factors together in computer programmes to allow doctors and patients to access an output number which describes the patient's estimated overall risk of an actual or future specific disease. This is clever and narrows down population statistics to more individualised factors, and provides the 'ballpark' figures for GPs to discuss with their patients.

On the down-side, risk scores do not represent every risk factor that a patient might have. They have also become so ubiquitous in general practice that they may become a substitute for thinking. Like other performance indicators, they act as a lever to standardising care. However, like all guidelines, they can leave GPs feeling that if they don't use them and their subsequent recommendations, they are at risk of criticism and complaint.

QRISK2 is a part of QoF for English GP income generation. As in any employment, GPs work to fulfil their contracts and since 2004, GMS GPs are partly paid for completing QoF in England (Wales and Scotland have recently retired their QoF indicators). The terms of QoF are published annually on the NHS Employers website and it is used also by many PMS practices. This book uses English GP QoF as examples. QoF breaks down detection, investigation, and management of a number of illnesses into points or indicators, to financially reward practices who are offering 'best practice' by showing that they have performed well, according to best medical evidence. QoF indicators are set by NICE and can alter to reflect different medical priorities over the years.

An example: (the *contractor is the GP practice) over management of hypertension would be:*

- *The contractor establishes and maintains a register of patients with hypertension*

This is a sensible ambition, to offer patients with hypertension good care. Also:

- *The percentage of patients with hypertension in whom the last blood pressure reading (measured in the preceding 12 months) is 150/90 mmHg or less*

Percentages are not set at 100%. Patients can refuse recommended therapy and not penalise the doctor financially as they are recorded under 'exemption recording'. In theory, there is no pressure to make patients comply to create income. However, lots of work is undertaken in practices, counting and recording activity. There is pressure to achieve QoF targets to maintain incomes comparable to other practices and recruit good standard medical staff. QoF allows the GP practice to align to NICE guidance and latest best medical evidence as reviewed by experts.

Within QoF are two risk scores CHA_2DS_2VASc and QRISK2.

CHA_2DS_2VASc helps decide the risk of future systemic embolism, usually an ischaemic stroke or transient ischaemic attack (TIA), in a patient who is in atrial fibrillation (AF).

QRISK2. In England this is used to determine a patient's 10-year cardiovascular risk of heart attack and stroke (CVD), but other risk tool scoring systems available are Framingham and the Joint British Society 3 (JBS3) risk scores.

Outside of QoF, a culture of risk scoring has emerged. On one hand risk scores may become a substitute for careful consultations and on the other they help stratify detected risk factors into a number in order to individualise and aid patient and clinician decisions. Examples of commonly used risk scores (again useful for GPs to have on their desktops) in primary care are as follows:

- CHA₂DS₂VASc to risk assess the likelihood of future systemic embolisation and so the recommendation for anticoagulation in people with nonvalvular AF
- HASBLED for the estimation of bleeding risk, used to risk-assess patients recommended for anticoagulation from their CHA₂DS₂Vasc score
- Wells score for deep vein thrombosis (DVT) and pulmonary embolism (PE) diagnosis
- Modified Early Waring Score (MEWS) or National Early Warning Score (NEWS) for detection of the severely ill patient
- CURB score for deciding on requirement to admit or not admit a patient with community-acquired pneumonia to hospital
- FeverPAIN Score or Centor Criteria to risk assess the possibility of strepto-coccus sore throats and subsequent requirement for antibiotics

Risk scores have become, on occasion, portals for hospital admission, regard-less of GP clinical opinion. They can be time consuming, especially if duplicating a history and examination, and GPs should know where to find them and what to do with them in an instant. This last item is a strength of risk scores. As the outcome is tightly defined, the recommended action is usually very clear.

Passing risk score information onto the patient requires GPs to invest in the risk assessment outcome as it is provided to us, to understand it and it's implications in depth. If GPs address the issues mentioned above they are a useful adjunct to decision making. Passing information on to patients should be by discussion but there are also Patient Decision Aids (PDAs), also called Shared Decision Aids. I find these most useful to GPs as well as the patients! These are the tables of 'smiley faces'. I recommend you enter QRISK2 into your search engine and input a well patient's (that is a primary prevention patient) details in and press submit. This might be yourself or a fantasy patient. The process is remarkably fast and you will read a risk over 10 years of possible CVD and see a PDA table:

Your risk of having a heart attack or stroke within the next 10 years is:

13.8%

In other words, in a crowd of 100 people with the same risk factors as you,
14 are likely to have a heart attack or stroke within the next 10 years.

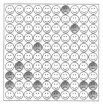

This table has been pasted using a fantasy patient at the QRisk2 site in 2017.

We will now look further in depth at the CVD risk score programme based on populations from England and Wales, QRISK2, in order to widen our thinking about risk factors. It can also be used in Scotland, N. Ireland, and internationally, though NHS Scotland also recommends ASSIGN, a Scottish population-derived risk tool. QRISK is integrated into the computer systems of all the major GP systems.

QRISK2: A RISK SCORE FOR THE PREDICTION OF CVD IN PRIMARY PREVENTION

There are four types of populations in primary care:

- Those with the illness already. GPs refer to treatment plans for them as secondary prevention; they are already unlucky in their health
- Those at high risk of the disease due to an amalgamation of risk factors; this is the group QRISK2 will try to identify.
- Those who are at low risk of the disease as they have low risk factor scores.
- Those who have one high risk variable which alone determines a high risk of this future illness and possible intervention, e.g. familial hypercholesterolaemia.

In 2014, NICE published guidance, *Cardiovascular disease: risk assessment and reduction, including lipid modification, clinical guideline 181.** This guideline recommends assessing our patient's risks of CVD and CVA by using QRISK2, which updates annually and is available at http://www.qrisk.org/ and can be freely accessed by anyone. NICE then uses QRISK2 scores to target cholesterol and hypertension therapy, using risk scores of 10% and 20% over 10 years of CVD respectively, as 'high risk' and recommend benefits of therapeutic intervention. NICE also recommends healthy lifestyle advice but everyone should get that anyway. QRISK2 assesses people aged 25–84 years old inclusive, selecting information about their

- Ethnicity
- Age
- Gender
- Family history of heart disease in a first degree relative (child, sibling or parent) below 60 years old

The above items cannot be changed by the patient. Then there are possibly modifiable items included which are

- Smoking status
- Systolic blood pressure

---

* Cardiovascular disease: risk assessment and reduction, including lipid modification. Clinical guideline 181 Published: 18 July 2014 at: https://www.nice.org.uk/Guidance/cg181.

- Ratio of total serum cholesterol/ high density lipoprotein cholesterol (HDL-C)
- Body mass index (BMI)
- Townsend deprivation score from national census which postcodes individuals for deprivation
- Treated hypertension
- Rheumatoid arthritis
- Chronic kidney disease (CKD)
- Type 2 diabetes (T2DM)
- AF

We will explore some features of genetics and epigenetics.

FAMILY HISTORY, ETHNICITY, GENES AND EPIGENETICS

QRISK2 asks the user to input a family history question:

Tick if a first degree relative (biological parent or sibling) has had cardiovascular disease below the age of 60 years old.

But what if two brothers had heart attacks at 62 years old? What if five brothers had heart attacks in their late 60s? Is that relevant? Of course, 'yes', but to calculate any algorithm there has to be cut-offs, i.e. values at which the tool decides significance. Be it an investigation, a history question, etc. a decision is made about levels of normal and abnormal, made by the algorithm makers, not the patient. GPs should listen to the patient and decide whether they fit the tool we are using. Patients all have cut-offs in our modern medical lives of information technology and statistics; here it is a family history of relevance in close relatives under 60 years old.

A 55-year-old man, non-smoker, with no other risk factors and no family history aged under 60 years, has a risk of developing CVD (angina, myocardial infarction [MI]), TIA or CVA of 6.9% over the next 10 years. Put it in at http://www.qrisk.org/ and check! This is virtually the average background risk at that age. This is important as nobody has *no* risk and anybody can develop serious illness despite having no obvious risk factors.

However, another man, aged 55 years old with no other risk factors except one relative who has had CVD below the age of 60 years old, has a QRISK2 estimate of 10.5%. Following the NICE primary prevention of CVD guidance this figure from QRISK2 of over 10% leads to a recommendation of offering him long-term statin prescriptions. Just a note here that QRISK2 refers to all strokes and although generally atheroma is associated with ischaemic CVA, hypertension may be associated with both ischaemic and haemorrhagic CVAs. The proportion of CVAs which are haemorrhagic though is low. The early studies of hypertension lowering therapy had the strongest primary outcome as CVA reduction and other preventions (heart disease, heart failure and renal disease) were less strongly correlated to reductions in blood pressure.

CVD is more prevalent amongst some racial groups than others. Asian Indians have a three to five times higher risk of CVD and are more likely to suffer their MIs at a younger age. There is an epidemic of CVD in Asia and many books and articles indicate that this is due to abnormal cholesterol and triglyceride levels (dyslipidaemia), hypertension, obesity, high salt intake, high fat intake and sedentary life styles. The economic development of affected countries has led people to live longer and, as CVD and CVA incidence increase with age. In addition, urban lifestyle adoption, including changes in diets and exercise, add to CVD risk.

Ethnicity alters the risk assessment of our population. The fastest growing group in the UK coming into the 25 plus age group are those of mixed race. How do patients describe themselves when their skin is light brown with two grandparents from Pakistan and two Caucasians from Newcastle? How much does the role of genes affect them? How diluted are diluted genes?

In a nutshell, risk scores are the best we can currently do and cannot capture all genes and their dilutions. Ethnicity relates to the 23 pairs of genes we carry around, look after and pass to our children. We know intuitively that some racial groups are more likely to be obese than others, but within a racial group one person may eat and exercise to the same degree as another but be more prone to obesity. Unravelling the understanding behind this is fascinating and uncertain.

The genome-wide association studies (GWAS) regularly report various genetic aberrations which make people prone to CVD. For some, it is a problem with a gene determining nitrous oxide (NO) at the endothelium, which acts usually as a vasodilator. For some, it is genetic tendencies to T2DM, or hypertension, or obesity. For others, it is a problem with a subtype of apoprotein which is important in lipoprotein regulation. Apoproteins were discovered in the 1970s and their subfeatures are now being unravelled. Some forms of apoprotein E genotypes are linked to higher LDL-C (low density lipoprotein-cholesterol) levels and to subsequent CVD.[*] In London, the LOLIPOP[†] (London Life Sciences Population) study has researched genetic variables in Londoners of South Asian ethnicity relating to T2DM, hypertension, obesity and CVD and identified a number of genetic changes which may make those individuals more at risk despite lifestyle issues. *Does genetics provide an easy answer then?*

No! There are scores of genes now associated with CVD. Unravelling those which are important and when is fascinating, and may ultimately lead to new therapeutic drugs individualised to the person's genetic makeup. Unfortunately, the simple identification of one or two major common genetic disorders ripe for targeting has not yet been achieved. We could follow the same line of evidence and thinking for obesity (about 135 genes have been linked to obesity so far),

---

[*] Khan TA, Shah T, Prieto D et al. Apolipoprotein E genotype, cardiovascular biomarkers and risk of stroke: Systematic review and meta-analysis of 14 015 stroke cases and pooled analysis of primary biomarker data from up to 60 883 individuals. *International Journal of Epidemiology* 2013;**42(2):**475–492.

[†] The LOLIPOP Study at: http://www.lolipopstudy.org/.

for T2DM, or for hypertension. As an aside, individualising patient medication according to genetics is now starting to occur, e.g. testing for thiopurine methyltransferase (TPMT) in patients before starting azathioprine. People who genetically lack or are deficient in TPMT are not prescribed azathioprine as their metabolism is different and they risk myelosuppression, bleeding, sepsis and death on the drug.

Is CVD risk related to the new science of epigenetics? Epigenetics* is a fast-growing science concerning the understanding of material inherited but which is not a fundamental part of our DNA. Epigenetic material can control gene expression and is common and complex. It appears that environment and lifestyle factors, e.g. diet, may create physical changes, such as methylation of DNA. This interacts with our genes and determines which gene sequences are suppressed and which are active. This effect may be lasting and transmissible through ourselves and our offspring. Through DNA methylation, histone modification, and non-coding RNA (ncRNA)-associated gene silencing, epigenetic change may occur to trigger or subdue particular genes. Methylation of DNA may occur through environmental factors occurring in the mother, e.g. maternal diet, and may then affect the embryo's DNA methylation and the future baby's genetic expression. Studies in mice have suggested that a high fat maternal diet may create obese mice offspring through epigenetic modification. Therefore, epigenetics may have a part to play in future risks of CVD that is not directly related to parental DNA but more to its suppression by epigenetic changes, some of which are environmental. Lifestyle and upbringing factors are also very important, but epigenetics is an independent risk to continuing obesity in the mice offspring. It is also postulated that changes in methylation of DNA may cause other effects, including cancer. Changes in dietary factors, like folic acid intake, may alter methylation rates in DNA so our diets may alter our epigenetics which in turn may influence our genetic expressions and subsequent disease tendencies. Deciding on a family history without considering epigenetic and also upbringing environmental factors may in the future be rather old fashioned.

Modifiable factors affecting CVD risk used in QRISK2 estimations are listed above. This book is not a text on clinical medicine and these factors are determined as important in CVD. Other factors not requested by QRISK2 but which may be relevant are alcohol intake, diet and exercise, independent of inputting BMI measurement.

Guidance for reducing risks of CVD once the patient has been counselled that he/she has a higher than recommended risk of CVD includes healthy diet and exercise. The NICE guideline committee searches systematically for evidence to base their lifestyle recommendations on. It is difficult to show primary prevention of CVD in patients who have taken up exercise or changed dietary habits to more fish, fruit and grains than their peers. There is no strong trial evidence that these lifestyle modifications prevent CVD. This may be due to

* Genomic imprinting at: http://www.geneimprint.com/site/what-is-imprinting.

the lack of funding for these trials compared to pharmaceutical development and marketing. This is unfortunate as the profits are better population health. However, exercise appears in the guidance as a positive recommendation and taken with benefits of socialisation, relaxation, increased muscle strength, reduction in certain cancer rates and prevention of CVD, it seems reasonable. It also fits intuitive GP physiology views of vasodilation through exercise being a protective factor. Possibly the changes from vasodilation to vasoconstriction help maintain vascular compliance and reactivity compared to prolonged vaso-constriction from inertia.

Recommendations for lifestyle benefits are arduous for a busy worker or carer. A patient may not want to change lifestyle and may be happy the way they are. If they do take on exercise, the recommended time is 150 minutes of moderate intensity aerobic exercise a week, or 75 minutes of vigorous aerobic exercise a week, or a mix. Or they may prefer muscle strengthening exercises twice a week. Although listed in the full guideline, it is unlikely that most GPs know which exercises sit in which recommendation. Anyhow, exercise becomes a usual part of daily routine in the guidance, in contrast with the car-based travel and computer-based work many people now do, including GPs. NICE also states that '*People should be advised to eat less than 30% of their total diet as fat of which 7% or less are saturated fats and cholesterol is less than 300 g a day.*' Few of us have any clear idea, GP or patient, how to calculate this at the supermarket and take-away shops, and dietary detail could be improved at many levels. For instance, how much fat is on a fish shop battered fish as a part of the day's total? In addition, '*People should replace saturated fats with monosaturated or polyunsaturated fats and use olive oils, rapeseed to cook and for spreads, wholegrain starches, reduce sugar including fructose, 5 portions of fruit and veg a day, 2 portions of fish, one of which is oily and 5 portions of unsalted nuts, seeds and legumes.*' This information is very difficult to follow when shopping and dietary publications need to be more available. However, there is no evidence of benefit for all-cause mortality for many of these dietary interventions.

For the GP, advice, guidance, risk tools and recommendations are helpful but not complete and we should still use expertise helping the patient understand risk and translating this into practical measures. Uncomfortably, where there is no evidence NICE has come down on the side of top-down medicine, telling the public what to do with no real proof in the areas concerned. Ballpark figures of benefit given as 0% proven benefit would be helpful in providing clinical honesty. It is tempting as a GP to intervene with medications. It grants us medical exper-tise and for some people will have great benefits. However, we are unable to very accurately pinpoint beneficiaries in a primary prevention population. Be aware that there are lots of exceptions and special cases, and we should read the guid-ance to understand these.

An in-depth analysis of statin therapy led NICE to support the use of ator-vastatin 20 mg for primary prevention of CVD, particularly as it had become cost effective and was shown to reduce the risk of non-fatal heart attacks in the population (but not fatal heart attacks and not all cause mortality). Patients aged 85 years old or over, and so outside the QRISK2 population group, are included as possibly benefiting from atorvastatin 20 mg od, although there have been no trials in this age group. Simvastatin had previously been preferred but the MHRA in 2012 informed doctors that there was an increased risk of myopathy due to interactions with simvastatin and amlodipine in liver enzyme metabolism, such that the maximum dose of simvastatin to be used is 20 mg with amlodipine. Dual prescriptions for hypertension and dyslipidaemia are common in the older age groups. Atorvastatin at 10 mg or 20 mg is much less likely to cause interactions with amlodipine in liver metabolism. In 2008, an MHRA Drug Safety Unit (DSU) update stated that statins may interact at liver metabolism with a number of medications, including erythromycin and clarithromycin, and the statin should be discontinued if on this medication. Smokers are more likely to have COPD and receive clarithromycin or erythromycin for chest infections and at the same time be on amlodipine for hypertension and a statin for dyslipidaemia and primary prevention of CVD. Guidelines often do not explore risks of polypharmacy and adverse drug reactions, interactions and side-effects. It is very difficult to find specific numbers of harms from medications online. A search on atorvastatin via the online Yellow Card reporting system at MHRA reveals many adverse reactions reported but they cannot all be proven as due to the medication. Whilst GPs want clarity, we must accept that it is difficult to prove certainty.

GPs, seeing 30–40 patients a day, and trying to enact the ensuing work from those interactions, some of which is on their computers to meet NHS organisational demands, are expected to know about new guidance and feel expert. The problem is that there are lots of journals but not one port of call to get this information and GPs undertake a lot of reading to try to keep up. If they don't keep up they would not know that some of the key changes in lipid modification set out in *Cardiovascular disease: risk assessment and reduction, including lipid modification, NICE clinical guideline 181 2014* might be abbreviated to the following:

- Cholesterol testing can be taken non-fasting rather than fasting.
- Risks of CVD considered worthy of medication were reduced to 10% 10-year risk.
- Atorvastatin 20 mg daily is preferred to simvastatin 40 mg a day.
- Primary hypercholesterolaemia might relate to a cholesterol over 7.5 mmol/L with a family history and those with a level over 9 mmol/L are recommended to be referred.
- Patients with kidney function eGFR <60 mls/min, or any albuminuria, should be on atorvastatin. But patients with eGFR <30 mls/min should be referred for a specialist opinion first.

NICE is a great site and 'NICE weekly updates', if you register for email updates, gives a list of new guidance. Unfortunately, much of it is of miniscule interest to GPs so it is difficult to capture a short update each week though there are strides being made in this direction. Perhaps the RCGP should be distilling the necessary guidelines for GPs and working with NICE to offer a single portal to updates. Certainly, advice would fit better with GP practice if modified by GPs. Reading through the full guideline gives an appreciation of the amount of work put into guideline development and most of us only refer to the short guidelines and recommendations.

Risk Aversion: Cultures and experiences

Despite knowing the evidence, clinicians and patients can become risk adverse due to personal experiences.

Scenario: Anaphylaxis after vaccination

The GP vaccinates baby Y at eight weeks old. Baby Y seemed well at the time but immediately after collapses with anaphylaxis and the GP institutes adrenaline and resuscitation. The baby has a stormy time as an IP and makes a slow recovery. The parents blame the GP for giving the vaccination. The GP is upset and anxious about the baby's anaphylaxis, hostility from the parents and possible complaint. The GP now avoids baby clinics, seeing newborns in clinic and reading about vaccinations. The GP knows that risks of anaphylaxis are 1 in 1,000,000 but having experienced one she no longer believes literature that states that vaccination is safe.

In 2008, there was an influenza H1N1 pandemic and unfortunately a few pregnant women developed severe symptoms, illness and some died. GPs and midwives were instructed to immunise pregnant women with the influenza vaccine and this is now standard practice. At the time, some GPs and many midwives were reluctant to take on this work as they had been trained not to immunise in pregnancy (they were risk averse). There were no long-term data on outcomes for mothers and babies before the programme was instituted. Due to the speed of the pandemic spread, there was no training and little explanation given for the change in practice but plenty of weekly guidance produced by PHE and RCGP. Some GPs had not given influenza injections for years as this had been delegated to practice nurses, which also complicated clinician attitudes and behaviour. Since the pandemic there has been concern that a small number of children may have developed narcolepsy from the Pandemrix vaccine, which is no longer used in pregnancy. However, the vaccination programme was very safe in general and influenza vaccination is now routinely given at any stage of pregnancy to protect the pregnant mother from flu.

Pertussis vaccination is also given in later pregnancy to protect the neonate, prior to routine baby vaccination, from whooping cough.

GPs require training, time and support to take on new practice, especially when there is a change in culture. Referring to non-adopters as 'risk averse' at meetings, as I have witnessed, is poor leadership and fails to recognise the complexity of primary care. To keep completely up to date, to read every GP journal and updating email from authorising bodies and educational sources is a full-time job in itself. GPs could become a very knowledgeable group who don't have any time to see patients! Being unable to access, absorb, understand, and assess all information creates a professional group who sometimes sit with both interest and cynicism.

Improving GPs' new skills and knowledge requires debate within the profession about how to achieve this. I recommend updated basic information within articles (online or in paper) routinely. As an example, an article on monoclonal antibody use in rheumatoid arthritis would have a small, boxed resource about monoclonal antibody actions. If done routinely this would mean that some new information would be absorbed by us over time as repeated exposure helps learning and skill development. This is also true of statistical truths. GPs are not statisticians and yet they are offered papers and guidelines to read which explore different methods of study and statistical outcomes in terms of sensitivity, specificity, significance(p), negative and positive predictive values (NPV and PPV), odds ratios (OR), relative and absolute risks (RR and AR), etc. Even if the basics of probability and confidence intervals (CI) are understood, the seemingly easiest papers will add a 'logistic regression' or some such to prevent full critical analysis of a study by most GPs. Statisticians are rarely listed as authors on papers and should be. We have no idea how many medical statisticians determine study designs in the UK. Again, structured revision statistical boxes would help GPs learn and refresh knowledge. Many GP articles already have useful outcome boxes, so I am suggesting an addition of a small revision box. Alternatively, learning modules on new physiology or statistics, or open access to assessment questions with model explanations could be developed. The RCGP curriculum is currently very wide, perhaps a more defined GP curriculum in which GPs are offered structured renewal and updates every 10 or 15 years of their career would help. To create knowledgeable GPs there should be investment in continued learning and development relevant to the GP curriculum with appropriate manageable time allocation.

PRESCRIBING ISSUES AND GUIDANCE INTEGRATION

Guidelines should be clear and synthesise with each other for primary care practitioners. Examples of possible confusion and pitfalls in practice are described below.

Drug names are poor. They do not usually reflect the use of the drug and brand names are not related to the generic name, which again has often no relevance to the action or use. Brand names are sometimes used on repeat prescriptions to align with government pressure to reduce costs if they are cheaper than prescribing generically. It would be less confusing if GPs prescribed generics and the use of cheap brands, or occasionally recommended same brand use, should sit with pharmacists in the pharmacy. As a minimum, the generic name should always be additionally printed on the patient direction label so the public know they are on the same medication. Often the pharmacy label obscures box print, which is tiny.

There are some medications for which errors are more common due to lack of clarity in names or packaging. A 2013 Drug Safety Unit* email highlighted risperidone and ropinirole as two similar names and a GP case of prescribing mercaptopurine instead of mercaptamine. Most GPs have not heard of mercaptamine and never prescribe it; it is in unfamiliar circumstances that mistakes happen. GPs should report to MHRA problems that occur in practice to highlight issues.

There is a traffic light system for drug prescribing and green medications refer to most medications, which are initiated and prescribed by GPs.

Orange medications are prescribed in a joint care manner with secondary care specialists initiating them and providing advice on monitoring the medication. An example would be starting methotrexate in a patient with rheumatoid arthritis in OPC. The GP practice performs and monitors the blood tests and issues the repeat prescriptions and the patient remains under occasional rheumatology OPC review.

The last group are red drugs. These drugs are those in which GPs are deskilled but which may cause problems and interactions for patients. Examples are chemotherapy agents, monoclonal antibodies, and HIV medications. Antiviral HIV medications have been used successfully for decades and yet GPs are still not prescribing these medications and gaining skills in this therapeutic area. Red drugs are prescribed and dispensed only in secondary care which deskills GPs and risks patient side-effects and harms in co-prescribing. There is an excellent, easy to access HIV checker[†] in which the GP can check their acute or repeat prescriptions against HIV medications.

Sometimes guidelines don't feel joined up. If a patient has a simple infection causing coughing, GPs are advised that this can last for three weeks. However, a cough that lasts over three weeks may bring the patient to the GP because they have read the 2016 PHE campaign message on early detection of lung cancer.[‡] 'If you've had a cough for three weeks or more, it could be a sign of lung disease, including cancer.' In the winter of 2016 some patients developed a flu-like illness followed by a hacking cough which lasted six to eight weeks before finally vanishing without antibiotics. Another guideline is the NICE lung cancer guidelines which suggest a CXR for lung cancer in an unexplained cough. Coughing weeks after a cold may not easily be explained but is not uncommon, so the guidelines sit uncomfortably beside each other. This can create over or under investigation and risk patient and GP anxiety. GPs may feel they have missed a long-term cough if they do not X-ray the chest and the patient ends up having a lung cancer. It seems that the bringing together of different guidelines and knowledge, which is the prerogative of the GP, requires more GPs to be working across system and expert boundaries to acknowledge the overlapping and grey areas of guidelines.

---

* Drug Safety Update 24 April 2013 at: https://www.gov.uk/drug-safety-update/recent-drug-name-confusion.

† HIV checker at: http://www.hiv-druginteractions.org/checker.

‡ 3 Be Clear on Cancer respiratory symptoms campaign 2016at: https://www.gov.uk/government/news/be-clear-on-cancer-respiratory-symptoms-campaign-launches.

NICE produced *Ovarian cancer: recognition and initial management Clinical guideline [CG122]*, published in April 2011. This important guideline introduced CA125 testing and USS for women with possible symptoms of ovarian cancer. NICE makes no mention of postmenopausal (PMB) or intermenstrual bleeding (IMB) as relevant symptoms in the guidance for primary care diagnosis and yet 15% of ovarian cancers may have these. I tried to check the algorithm at the end of the short clinical guideline for information on IMB but on clicking through this it led to the full guideline. The full guideline site did not immediately yield the algorithm, by which time interest was lost and I abandoned my search. In June 2015 *Suspected cancer: recognition and referral NICE guideline [NG12]* was published, pasting the same symptoms over from the ovarian cancer guideline and again not mentioning IMB or PMB as possible symptoms of ovarian cancer. This sparked my interest again. Ovarian cancer does not appear as a cause in the *Heavy Menstrual Bleeding: assessment and management* clinical guideline from NICE, and as it may occasionally cause abnormal bleeding I expected some reference would be made to it somewhere. Back to the original ovarian cancer guideline then and the full NICE ovarian cancer guideline states: *'Despite the fact that abnormal vaginal bleeding was linked with the existence of ovarian cancer* (Hamilton et al. 2009; Goff et al. 2007) *the GDG felt that the urgent clinical pathway already established for abnormal vaginal bleeding (NICE, 2005) was likely to detect ovarian cancer as part of that investigation. Therefore, they did not include this symptom in the recommendations.'* The 2005 guideline is no longer easily available on the NICE website and anyway, no GP expects to jump from one set of guidance to another to find best practice. My message is persistent and urgent; make guidelines usable! I am also asking you, our readers as interested clinicians, to get involved in a small way as guideline developers or reviewers.

Patients also look for information online. Some admit that they become neurotic reading about their symptoms as all online sites highlight serious adverse possibilities to avoid falsely reassuring patients. Many read newspaper and magazine articles or watch health TV programmes. Some cut out articles and bring them in to update their GP! Patients therefore may attend without a full picture yet sure in their knowledge, which can be difficult to manage. They may be biased according to their own experiences or those of their families and friends. GPs are no different. If we don't like a finding or it doesn't fit our own experience then we are likely to reject it or at least have more difficulty taking on the change in practice.

Useful resources:

- The National Institute for Health and Care Excellence (NICE) at https://www.nice.org.uk/
- Scottish Intercollegiate Guidelines Network (SIGN) at http://www.sign.ac.uk/
- NHS Evidence at https://www.evidence.nhs.uk/
- MHRA and DSU and https://yellowcard.mhra.gov.uk/

- British National Formulary (BNF) at https://orchid.medicinescomplete.com/about/publications.htm?pub=bnf

Medical Statistics: A brief introduction

Assessing evidence makes most GPs groan because they think back to the times of journal clubs as undergraduates! There are few GPs who are expert in medical statistics but that skill is not actually needed when it comes to evidence appraisal. GPs need an inquisitive mind and a process to simply assess the key aspects of the paper.

The fear of not being able to do evidence appraisal often puts very good clinicians off commenting. It also allows the growth of poor studies, as they are not critically assessed by as many clinicians as we would like. Lack of evidence appraisal also increases cynicism amongst those who are told that a study should change behaviour when they cannot be sure of the evidence for doing so. Most clinicians are not on sure ground when working out advantages and disadvantages of trial design, and dealing with terms such as p, CI, standard deviations (SD), AR, and RR and in recent years this has been more widely acknowledged by experts.

STANDARD DEVIATION, ABSOLUTE RISK AND RELATIVE RISK

Standard deviation

Scenario: Outlying test result and normal distribution

Mr Y attends for his blood tests results and has been asked to attend early due to a high prostate specific antigen (PSA), which he has checked annually. He attends his regular GP because 'he has been through all this before'. He has had a prostate biopsy twice which has been negative and his PSA has not altered over 10 years. His urologist discharged him to his GP for surveillance and recommended annual recheck and re-referral if the PSA level increased. That was five years ago. In this case Mr Y's PSA of 6.1 ng/ml was outside of the laboratory determined normal value of less than 4 ng/ml but the same as usual for him.

It is usual to take 2 standard deviations (2SD) from the mean as a cut off for defining normality as this distribution will cover 95% of the population. This though will allow 2.5% of the normal public to have an outlying figure at either end of the normal range (5% in total). That is, 2SD accounts for 95% of the variation in figures from the mean and if 2SD has been used for the test then Mr Y just happens to be in the higher 2.5% (assuming a 2SD cut-off lab test value). The upper 2.5% of PSA results in the normal population will overlap with the population who have a high PSA due to prostate cancer. This has led to Mr Y having two prostate biopsies, both negative. However, after establishing him as having a 'high-normal PSA', it is difficult to find a mechanism to prevent repeated 'rediscovery'.

Study results can be presented in a variety of ways. Over a few years, the realisation that RR reporting can be misleading has led authors and clinicians to encourage the use of AR when presenting the magnitude of harms and benefits of therapies as RR can make benefits appear bigger than they really are.

Example: Absolute risk versus relative risk: different ways of presenting risk
In a study, drug D was tested to see whether it could prevent pneumonia in people over five years. One thousand people were given drug D, and 1000 people were given a matching placebo for five years. The two groups were matched for age, sex, asthma, COPD, smoking, etc., so variables appeared to be fairly distributed throughout the two study arms. Let's assume at five years there are no patients who dropped out of the study and let's also assume no harms from drug D.

The result was:
Placebo group: 150 people (15%) developed pneumonia by the end of the study. Drug D group: 100 people (10%) developed pneumonia.

Absolute numbers

In this case, the benefit of drug D in absolute terms is 15%–10% = 5% fewer people developed pneumonia while on drug D than on the placebo.

The 5% is considered the absolute risk reduction (ARR).

Relative numbers

However, this difference can be presented in a different way.

15% of people developed pneumonia on the placebo and 10% on drug D, so the improvement can also be stated as a 33% relative risk reduction (RRR) in pneumonia due to drug D because 10% is 33% less (or 1/3) than 15%.

A 33% RRR in pneumonia due to drug D is a correct number but it looks much more appetising than when we use the absolute numbers which is one of the reasons why relative numbers are used if we wanted to sell drug D!

The trial might also be of interest because it showed that even with no treatment 85% of people did not get pneumonia. Suddenly the choices about taking medication D become more difficult.

For some people, it may highlight that even with the drug D 10% of people still got pneumonia and only 5% fewer than with the placebo, so 95% of people would take the drug for five years for no benefit. These people might wonder what harms they might incur and whether they can be bothered to take a tablet.

Clearly how numbers are presented to readers in conjunction with the risk of an individual getting an underlying disease becomes important and sways decisions. If a patient has a disease already they may well opt for treatment, providing the harms of the medication are acceptable. If a well person has a higher risk of developing a disease in the future they may well opt for preventive treatment too. However, in preventing a disease over a population, the commonality (prevalence) of the disease may dictate how people feel about taking preventive therapies and influence how public health bodies make decisions about benefits and costs of prevention.

CHANGES IN PREVALENCE OF CONDITIONS INFLUENCES STATISTICAL BENEFITS/HARMS

1. Disease M is an awful fatal disease affecting young people.

   Suppose disease M is present in 2 people out of a population of 10,000 (0.02% prevalence of disease M). Also suppose drug E prevents disease M developing in 50% of future sufferers because it is fantastic.

   Using the above information, the benefit of drug E will be to 1 in 10,000 of the population. That is, 0.01% of the population will benefit from therapy.

   10,000 people will take the medication and yet one person will develop the disease anyway, but due to drug E, one will stay healthy.

   It is unlikely that people will all take drug E as it will be highly unlikely to benefit them and may cause side-effects, inconvenience, and it will also be expensive to the NHS, possibly preventing affordability of other medications.

2. Suppose disease M is very common though and is present in 2 in 10 of the population (20% prevalence of disease M).

   Now asking the population to all take drug E to prevent the onset of disease M in 50% of potential sufferers will mean that its benefit will be to 1 in 10 of the population. 10 people will take drug E and one will still develop the disease and one will remain healthy.

   If the disease is very serious and drug E is harmless then, as everyone will know someone with disease M, it is likely that the medication will be accepted by people.

3. Postnatal screening of infants at day five has been extended in the last few years to include some very rare but high risk conditions, like Maple Syrup Urine Disease. Here the cost of universal neonatal testing is worthwhile because of the serious but preventable disability that is simply prevented by special diet and supplements for the handful of affected babies detected each year. Most GPs never see a case but there are also a small number of GPs each year who will have a case born into their practice list.

So, benefits, harms and costs of therapies will depend on the prevalence of the disease or condition, as well as the success of therapy and the seriousness of the condition. Immediately we start to weigh up benefits and harms against resource allocation, including skills, time and costs.

SENSITIVITY AND SPECIFICITY

Sensitivity and specificity are commonly-used terms and most GPs understand that figures nearest to 100% for each are best. They are commonly confused and yet their figures determine use of investigations frequently in medicine.

A true positive result (TPos) is one in which the positive test picks up the condition accurately, e.g. a 100% accurate test for the Y chromosome would pick up 100% of genetic men.

A false negative (FNeg) result is one in which the test is negative but the index case does have the condition, e.g. this would be high if the assay was not very accurate so that a genetic man tests negative for the Y chromosome.

A false positive result (FPos) is one in which the test is positive but the index case does not have the condition, e.g. a positive Y chromosome test in a genetic female. This rate would be zero for our 100% accurate assay.

A true negative result (TNeg) is one in which the test is negative and the case does not have the condition, e.g. genetic women would have 100% true negative testing for the Y chromosome.

Sensitivity is high if a test correctly rules in the diagnosis for people who have the condition and doesn't leave anyone with the disease out. Ideally all the positive results are True Positives and there are no False Negative results.

The number of patients who will have the condition is the number of True Positives and the number of False Negatives combined, so sensitivity is calculated simply as

TPos/(TPos+FNeg)

Example numbers:
Using a 100% accurate test for Y chromosome to detect genetic men we expect no false negative tests and all genetic men to test positive for the Y chromosome. Sensitivity would be 100%.

100 population of 50 men and 50 women tested for Y chromosome with 100% accurate assay:

TPos = 50 and FNeg = 0

50/(50+0) x100/1 = 100%

The PSA is not used as a national screening test because at the cut-off points recommended, it misses an unacceptable number of prostate cancers due to false negative tests and so, has low sensitivity.

Specificity is high if the test accurately rules out the disease correctly in healthy people; so the higher the figure, the less likely people who have not got the index condition will have a positive test. This rules out False Positive results and subsequent further investigation of fit people. Good specificity of a test will mean that most people have True Negative tests and as the population of fit people may contain True Negative and False Positive results specificity is calculated simply as

TNeg/(TNeg+FPos)

Example numbers:
In testing a population for genetic males using a test for the Y chromosome then we do not expect any True Negative results and we do not expect any women to test positive for the Y chromosome so False Positives should be zero for our assay. Therefore, specificity will be high at 100%.

100 population of 50 men and 50 women tested for Y chromosome with 100% accurate assay

TNeg=50 women and FPos= 0 women

50/(50+0) x100/1 =100%

PSA is not used as a screening test for prostate cancer because it has low specificity and unfortunately many men will have a raised PSA, perhaps due to urinary tract infection or prostatitis, and undergo a transrectal ultrasound scan (USS) of prostate and multiple prostatic biopsies only to be told they have no cancer and that they have had a false positive PSA result due to the low specificity of the test.

To improve sensitivity and specificity a number of tests or/and symptoms can be added together, to create a more accurate risk score. An example of this aggregation of statistics is in assessment of investigations for ovarian cancer as described in *NICE Ovarian cancer: recognition and initial management Clinical guideline [CG122] Published date: April 2011.* This guideline recommends the use of CA125 in ovarian cancer detection. The NICE clinical guideline* states:

- *Measure serum CA125 in primary care in women with symptoms that suggest ovarian cancer*
- *If serum CA125 is 35 IU/ml or greater, arrange an ultrasound scan of the abdomen and pelvis*

In the guideline, CA125 for the detection of ovarian cancer is used only in conjunction with symptoms to improve the specificity and sensitivity of testing. Symptoms of ovarian cancer can be very vague, such as abdominal bloating. NICE makes evidence on symptoms and tests for ovarian cancer freely available on its website and their statements are in italics below.

NICE evidence on detection of ovarian cancer from the symptom of *abdominal bloating*:

- *Sensitivity: 5% to 68%* **Sensitivity** *is the proportion of women with ovarian cancer who experienced the symptom in the year prior to diagnosis.*

This is wide variation fits with the subtle and variable symptoms which women with ovarian cancer might present within the year before the ovarian cancer diagnosis. Even the top figure of 68% of women in a study complaining of abdominal distension has a low True Positive rate. So, significant numbers

---

of women without abdominal distension will have ovarian cancer and high False Negatives.

- *Specificity: 62% to 98% **Specificity** is the proportion of women without ovarian cancer who did not experience the symptom within the last year.*

There is wide variability of symptoms among women who do not have ovarian cancer. Therefore there are a number of women who have abdominal distension symptoms but who do not have ovarian cancer, False Positive test.

To improve sensitivity of symptoms and testing to detect ovarian cancer, NICE then added in the use of CA125 and USS testing and derived the following figures:

Using figures from Hamilton et al. (2009) and Bankhead et al. (2005), approximately 0.23% of women with symptoms consistent with ovarian cancer in primary care actually have ovarian cancer. If all women with symptoms were referred to secondary care, around 1 in every 500 women referred would turn out to have ovarian cancer.

If women were only referred if they had a positive serum CA125 test or ultrasound scan, then 1 in every 157 referred would have ovarian cancer; 3% of women with ovarian cancer and symptoms would not be referred.

If women were only referred when both the CA125 test and ultrasound were positive, then 1 in every 26 referred would have ovarian cancer.

This is the pathway which was decided.

POSITIVE AND NEGATIVE PREDICTIVE VALUES

The **positive predictive value (PPV)** is the probability that a patient with a positive result does have the index disease.

As NICE states in its ovarian cancer guideline: 'The PPV of a given symptom for ovarian cancer is the proportion of women with that symptom who have ovarian cancer. For example, if a symptom had a PPV of 0.2% for ovarian cancer, 1 in 500 women with that symptom would have ovarian cancer. The PPV of a symptom for ovarian cancer in those presenting to primary care depends both on the sensitivity/specificity of the symptom and the background risk of ovarian cancer in this population. PPV: 0.01% to 0.30%'

In the NICE evidence for PPV above the highest PPV of abdominal distension of 0.3% translates into a risk of ovarian cancer for 1 in 300 women complaining of abdominal bloating. GPs know that abdominal bloating is a common symptom of weight gain, constipation, food intolerance, irritable bowel syndrome, etc. so a variable number of non-ovarian cancer sufferers are going to complain of distension; False Positive results.

The **negative predictive value (NPV)** of a result expresses the probability that the negative result correctly represents those without the index disease.

As the NICE ovarian cancer guideline says:

The NPV of a given symptom for ovarian cancer is the proportion of women without that symptom who do not have ovarian cancer. NPV: 99.95% to 99.98%.

In the NPV by NICE above, most women without abdominal distension do not have ovarian cancer. Given the low prevalence of ovarian cancer amongst women, this is not surprising.

I could not do better than quote NICE's work here to illustrate PPV and NPV. When GPs refer women, there are those with an obvious mass and symptoms in which the GP is almost certain that there is an ovarian cancer. There are also women in whom the symptoms are so nebulous that the possibility of cancer is much more remote and the statistics above help to quantify this. There are patients with a CA125 just above the 35iu cut-off for abnormal test or who have a mild abnormality on USS such as 'a small amount of free fluid in the abdomen.' There are women with a very high CA125, in the high hundreds perhaps, and/or a USS declaring a large suspicious solid ovarian mass. The statistics overall though suggest that those women with vague symptoms and some abnormality of CA125 and USS have an overall risk of ovarian cancer of 1 in 26. This information may be shared with our patients, depending where on the sliding scale of clinical diagnosis we have judged them and may prevent overwhelming anxiety in the lead up to assessment for patients.

GP tests which have a high specificity and sensitivity nearer to 100% are usually those using a type of genetic fingerprinting. An example of this is chlamydia testing by NAAT (nucleic acid amplification test) in which specificity and sensitivity lie above 94%. In one study* Combo 2 assay results were compared with the patient infected status, which were available through using other commercial NAATs. Sensitivity and specificity for Chlamydia trachomatis were 94.2% and 97.6%, respectively, in endocervical swabs. This study is dated 2003 and the reader will be aware that self-taken vaginal swabs for women with possible chlamydia infection is now recommended, unless the GP wants to also view the cervix or discharge.

This NAAT test for chlamydia has a sensitivity of 94.2%.

94.2% of people with a positive chlamydia test will have chlamydia. Unfortunately, 5.8% of people will have a False Negative test but still have chlamydia.

This NAAT test for chlamydia has a specificity of 97.6%.

97.6% of people who do not have chlamydia will not have a positive chlamydia test. Good. The higher the specificity the more likely a positive test means the disease or condition is present but it is not 100%. Unfortunately, 2.4% of people tested in this study will have a positive result but will not have chlamydia: this is a 2.4% False Positive result.

It is up to the GP to decide how many statistics they want to use in information analysis but I hope you have a grasp of the essentials and variability. Like all

* Gaydos CA, Quinn TC, Willis D et al. Performance of the APTIMA Combo 2 assay for detection of *Chlamydia trachomatis* and *Neisseria gonorrhoeae* in female urine and endocervical swab specimens. *Journal of Clinical Microbiology* 2003 January;**41(1):** 304–309.

skills, it requires practice and repetition to become competent and having understood the principles, it may be reasonable to trust respected resources.

We can now balance truth, as we see and assess it, better for our patients when discussing management plans. So far in this book we have thought about relevant laws and regulations that we bring into the consultation and we have skilfully collected our patient's information. Now we have used our knowledge and evidence base to consider the patient's problems and management. In the next section, we will explore the ethics and behaviours we bring with us into our consultations.

Useful resources:

- GetTheDiagnosis.org: A Database of Sensitivity and Specificity including an online calculator at: http://getthediagnosis.org
- The NNT site presents numbers needed to treat or harm in numbers or percentages at: http://www.thennt.com/
- How to critically appraise a paper in 10 minutes by James McCormack at: https://therapeuticseducation.org/sites/therapeuticseducation.org/files/Ten _Minute_Critical_Appraisal_of_an_RCT.pdf
- How to Read a Paper: The Basics of Evidence Based Medicine (Book) by Trisha Greenhalgh

4

Ethics and behaviours

Pupil: *I see an impassable gorge between what I truly feel (and so would naturally like to do) and what I know I should do, or am allowed to do. I think I am going to fall into the gorge and fail.*

Tutor: *Learning to fly can be useful.*

Pupil some years later: *I have learned to fly over gorges and become successful but now I see a huge mountain between my professional practice and what I think is ideal.*

Tutor: *Remember your flying principles; a mountain is just an upside-down gorge.*

This section on ethics and behaviours explores Aristotle's ethical model as a framework with which to develop ourselves as professionals. The Beauchamps–Childress ethical framework is discussed as an aid to critically analysing clinical scenarios and wider medical practice. GPs undertake a plethora of roles and act as role models, teachers and trainers, leaders and team members and relevant skills and pitfalls are discussed. GPs teaching within the consultation, balancing patient and learner needs, is an interesting area and also discussed in this section. GPs and their patients may bring cultural and religious factors into the consultation and the impact of these is explored.

As always, this section is a guide and does not direct the reader but facilitates awareness and options to improve self, clinical practice and medical practice more widely.

Ethical models

ARISTOTLE ETHICS

Although Aristotle lived a long time ago, in ancient Greece, he was a polymath of his time. Conclusions he came to concerning human ethics are still pertinent today.

First though, what is an ethic? It is a principle which determines the morality of our lives and how we want to behave. We all have attitudes and these determine our behaviours. Attitudes are developed initially by the interactions of personality and experiences. Using our personal, ethical codes modifies our innate attitudes and modifies how we behave. Sometimes, there can be conflict between the ethical codes we develop and the ethics of the group to which we belong, and by which we should abide. So, a set of ethical principles can be given to groups of people to set out how they should behave within their setting.

Medical professionals have a set of medical ethics. This set of principles will vary across the world, according to the ethical precepts of that country. When ethics are considered highly important, or a mandatory activity, they become rules and laws. GPs have their personal ethical codes, the ethical code of their profession and the laws and regulations which they should follow. The General Medical Council (GMC) has several guidelines on ethics but the overarching ethical principle which will sustain our careers is, not surprisingly, the first one in *Duties of a Doctor*:

'Make the care of your patient your first concern'.

Note that it doesn't say 'make sure you do what the patient wants as your first concern'. This is about best medical care. As soon as we become interested in ethical principles, we become self-aware. Behaviour is often, but not always, the visible result of our attitudes. We define attitudes ourselves, using our inner personality strengths and weaknesses and our cultural experiences. We are influenced by our societal values and laws, our culture, religion, friendships, families, school and work experiences. We will look at some religious and cultural variations amongst patients and GPs who are Catholic, Jewish and Muslim further along. GPs with strict religious views may find that they are in ethical conflict with some common UK medical practices. Patients with the same religious or cultural ethical codes will face the same problems, e.g. over abortion law, death rituals or family planning. Once we recognise outer influences on our lives and inner attitudes, we can free ourselves up to develop choice. This choice is self-improvement. Some people never develop it and never mature; they act to their childhood strengths throughout their lives, with varying degrees of success. Through self-actualisation, we learn to make decisions about whether we want to act the bully, the shouter, the taker or whether we want to be givers, listeners, lovers or carers. We can decide if we want risk, security, friendship, close colleagues and consciously decide whether we need to improve to gain these. We can decide whether we want to think well of ourselves and have self-confidence, whether we want to be over-confident or insecure and lacking in self-worth. We can decide to take ethical stances across our personal and professional lives or separate them. Ethics lead to self-improvement throughout our short lives.

Aristotle believed that the route to happiness lay in self-improvement. He described inherent traits or personality types as 'virtues' but this has such a starchy sound to it nowadays that I have relabelled them, with apologies to Aristotle, as behaviour(s). This is a colloquial use, and we mustn't forget that behaviour is the outward action of our decided attitudes. Behaviours have a variety of responses and Aristotle believed that good behaviour and happiness lies in avoiding the extremes. For instance:

One person is a coward, another rash and reckless. The optimum behaviour is courage.

One person is unkind sometimes cruel, another over-saccharine. The optimum behaviour is brotherly love.

One person is ignorant, another opinionated. The optimum behaviour is knowing wisely.

One person is mean and miserly, another over-giving and cloying. The optimum behaviour is generosity.

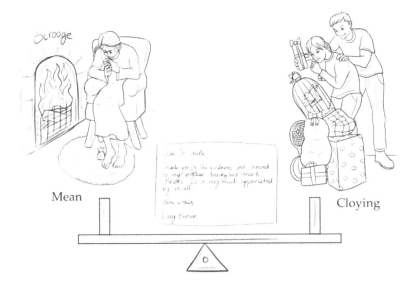

Think about your own inherent personality traits, the excesses of them as behaviours and where you lie within the scale.

- Do you like what you see?
- Is your behaviour effective?
- Are you happy with your performance or do you want or/and need to take steps to improve?
    – That's insight.

To gain insight, we must know ourselves, know what our alternatives are and recognise our blind spots. To achieve improvement, we sometimes need to understand why we respond as we do. Often it is through childhood, learned experiences. Sometimes, it is through very strong personality traits. To change we need to learn from our mistakes and failures and practice improvements repeatedly. In this way, we improve subconsciously and enjoy the person we have become. We discuss learning from failure further on.

A person brought up in a household of smacking may react by smacking and it will take some practice and correction to achieve a more meritorious response. Their aggressive behaviour is fuelled by learnt attitudes of anger or bullying. The other extreme to this would be someone who responds to any disagreement, however trivial with fear and timidity, perhaps bursting into tears at the first sign of being asked to do something. The person wanting to improve needs to practice control and develop calm.

We should ask:

- Have we done ourselves or others injustice?
- Have we offered a positive experience to ourselves and others?

In medical education, GPs have acted as experts and role models to generations of medical students and postgraduate trainees so this is very important and we explore this below in a look at the apprentice model of medical education.

BEAUCHAMPS–CHILDRESS FRAMEWORK FOR MEDICAL ETHICS

The Beauchamps–Childress model of medical ethics is the model most commonly taught in UK medical schools and comprises four principles which provide a framework for analysing ethical problems:

1. **Respect for autonomy:** Acting to let the patient make the best decision for themselves at that time and in that health context.
2. **Beneficence:** Acting in the best interests of the patient in order to do good.
3. **Non-maleficence:** Acting in the best interests of the patient to do no harm.
4. **Justice:** Acting in the best professional manner to distribute health care resources in a fair manner.

Medical problems are described below to illustrate the different principles but in fact all four principles are at work in each case.

Autonomy

Scenario: Acute appendicitis

A 19-year-old man attends the GP with a day's history of abdominal pain. It kept him awake in the night and now he is nauseated and feels sick. The pain has settled over McBurney's point, suggesting localised peritonitis over the appendix. The GP informs the patient of the findings, diagnosis and possible adverse outcomes. The patient exerts his autonomy and agrees to emergency admission for treatment. He undergoes early operation and recovers well.

In this case, the medical ethics are straightforward – GP and patient agree on strategy and there is a good outcome.

Scenario: Refusal to allow a referral with cancer

Mr Y, 28 years old, attends with a chesty cough. On auscultating his chest, the GP notices a lesion on the back of his chest which looks like a superficial spreading malignant melanoma. The GP mentions the finding and possible diagnosis and wants to refer him on a 2 week cancer (2WW) referral. Mr Y refuses and is adamant that he doesn't need referral.

This is upsetting for the doctor who has found what may be an early curable cancer, but the patient refuses to be referred. The first approach to making ethical decisions is to ensure that all the facts are known. In this case, there was no underlying situation mitigating against referral. As an adult with capacity, Mr Y is entitled to refuse referral and die of his untreated malignant melanoma. Autonomy tends to take priority in UK medical decision making.

In this instance, the GP explained the problem, gave him the British Association of Dermatology patient information leaflet (PIL) on melanoma and took a picture for him with his camera phone so he could see it. An appointment was agreed, with difficulty, for Mr Y to return the next week with a friend or his partner, or to see another doctor. He returned with his partner and agreed to referral.

Had Mr Y not done so then the sensible action for the doctor would have been to discuss the case at a practice meeting with the practice partners, managers and nurses and to ensure the records were clear. The GP would send a written letter to the patient outlining the concern and offering a future appointment at any time and would inform his defence body, who could offer further advice. If this young man had not returned and had subsequently died of this illness then the family may have complained against the GP. Clear pathways of attempted care are important, including recording of assessment of his capacity.

Beneficence and non-maleficence

Scenario: Heart attack but patient won't 'go in'

Mrs X is 76 years old and calls for a visit with chest pain. She refuses an ambulance so the GP visits. The pain sounds like a heart attack, which occurred the night before. There was associated visceral pain symptoms of sweating, nausea and dizziness with referred pain as a left arm ache. Now she feels improved and has a mild but persistent, tight chest pain.

In this case, Mrs X's capacity needs to be checked, as being unwell she may have a temporary loss of capacity. The GP explained to her that she had almost certainly had a myocardial infarction and that it was best practice to arrange her admission and that she might be suitable for primary percutaneous coronary intervention with angiography and stent (PPCI). The benefits of admission in the first 48 hours of myocardial infarction to prevent or act on acute dysrhythmia and the benefits to angina pain of PPCI were set out. In this case, it is very difficult to give patient's accurate ball park figures and this is discussed in the knowledge and evidence section of this book. However, it is honest to tell her that over 80% of patients will not die of their heart attack but that we cannot identify accurately who might become very ill or die. Finding ball park figures on home care in a 'treatment-by-PPCI' driven society is very difficult. Comparing figures to those of the 1970s may be biased by historical smoking rates (numbers of cigarettes were often 40–60 a day) and poverty rates, which are different to today's populations.

Harms for Mrs X would revolve mainly around bleeding rates if she did have PPCI intervention and would need to be compared to starting her on aspirin and clopidogrel in the community.

For Mrs X, the perceived harm was in leaving the security of her home. She felt that she would function much better at home and was aware that she could change her mind or call 999 at any time. Mrs X didn't want to leave home and felt intuitively that she was improving. The GP explored her home situation (a widow with a local supportive daughter who visited each week at least) and health views. During checking her mental capacity, there was an awkward moment when the GP asked, 'Can you tell me what might be the worst thing that happens to you if you stay at home?'

Mrs X looked at the GP patiently, 'You have already told me I might die, I know that, but I won't.'

In this situation, the patient had weighed up the benefits and harms of admission and used her autonomy to stay at home. She let the GP give 300 mg of soluble aspirin and tried a glyceryl trinitrate (GTN) spray with some benefit (BP was 120/78). She allowed the GP to phone her daughter to outline the problem. The daughter was supportive of her mum's decision and the GP. Mrs X had blood taken, refused travel to the practice for an electrocardiogram (ECG) or for outpatient clinic (OPC) or cardiac rehabilitation but took it easy for a week and started on secondary prevention medications long term. The GP visited the next day and a few more visits over weeks and the patient did very well. In this situation, a secondary medical management plan was created which was acceptable to her.

Scenario: The raccoon prevents admission
It is a rainy evening and a home visit is to a 35-year-old man with poorly controlled diabetes. He is thirsty and dizzy. A test of his urine reveals glycosuria and ketonuria – confirming diabetic ketoacidosis. He had a home capillary blood glucose measurement kit which measures 'Hi' when the GP tests his finger capillary glucose level. A read of the instructions with the machine reveals that 'Hi' blood capillary glucose equates to capillary glucose levels of 33 mmol/L or above! He is not confused, demonstrates capacity and refuses referral to hospital.

The first action again is to collect all the facts.

It transpires that he has no friends or family, and has a raccoon, which he won't leave. The GP suggests that the raccoon is taken to an animal sanctuary overnight and this can be arranged by social services and the GP as an emergency so that he won't worry.

The harm of real risk of death from diabetic ketoacidosis is discussed and the benefits of hospital admission to himself in the short and long term, and ultimately to his raccoon. He lights up a cigarette and refuses admission. An alternative plan is created. He agrees to drink plenty of very dilute squash and increase his evening insulin by 6 units and re-monitor his capillary glucose. He is told to re-contact the out-of-hours (OOH) GP if his condition worsens or call 999. The next morning the visit message is passed on to his GP who visits early, arranges his raccoon a place in a sanctuary via the social service department and Mr Y is admitted to a good outcome.

Justice

Justice often revolves around costs of procedures in society and how the NHS budget can be managed fairly. It is usually left to higher economic and ethical bodies to draw up guidance to help improve justice, e.g. NICE deciding whether a new tyrosine kinase inhibitor anticancer drug should be funded which improves patient life expectancy by 4 months against perhaps a desire to improve public health by spending on weight loss clinics to reduce obesity rates. At a local level, GPs relate to the individual patient and act as their advocate in most instances. Occasionally requests for care may be determined by GPs to be unjust and they may make a clinical decision using justice as their main determinant. However, if patients challenge the decision a second opinion should be sought.

Scenario: GP refuses an operation

Miss X is 18 years old and attends the GP wanting her right breast increased because it is smaller than the left and this is making her very miserable. On examination, the GP finds that the size difference is barely noticeable and explores the patient's concerns and mental state. The young woman is not depressed or at risk of self-harm but is adamant that she requires breast enhancement. The GP refuses with a reasonable explanation. The patient returns a few weeks later to make the same request in a more forceful manner. At this point, the GP refers her for a second opinion, which supports the GP's medical view of normal variation.

Using ethical models

The common scenario of starting warfarin or not in a patient is used to illustrate analysis of a case using all four ethical frameworks. Other scenarios relate to personal ethical values of truth telling or deceit.

Scenario: Using ethical frameworks to decide best therapy

Mrs X, 78 years old, attends the surgery and tells her GP that she has stopped her warfarin. This anticoagulant was started a year before due to onset of atrial fibrillation (AF) with a raised risk of systemic embolization (possibly stroke). She says she 'was never happy to be on it and yet didn't want to let down her cardiology specialist'. Having stopped it 6 weeks previously she had continued to feel well but had become very anxious over her decision. She had developed nausea, mild weight loss and insomnia. She described her anxiety as being about 'what if?'

The GP needs to establish that Mrs X has capacity to make decisions and her views on tablets, check-ups, anticoagulant monitoring on warfarin versus newer anticoagulants not requiring regular monitoring. Also, information should be collected on her symptoms and views on risks of stroke. Having gained all the facts, the GP should facilitate the patient to look at the benefits (beneficence) of anticoagulation. For Mrs X, this was calculated on this occasion as a risk of embolus of 12% against the harms of therapy (non-maleficence). On this occasion harm was calculated as a risk of 4.7% of major haemorrhage. These risks were calculated using CHA_2DS_2CVASc and HASBLED risk scores. The justice is that this lady should be offered anticoagulation (and different anticoagulants should be discussed) as this would be normal good practice in the United Kingdom. However, Mrs X has a right to exercise her autonomy and decide to restart, or not to restart, her anticoagulant. What were Mrs X's 'what ifs?' She was concerned that not taking anticoagulants would alienate her from her specialist, her GP and practice staff. She was concerned that if she had a stroke or transient ischaemic attack (TIA), there would be an element of blame from her family, friends, herself and the medical profession. She was concerned that she couldn't change her mind. The role of the GP was to set out the facts and explain possible risks and harms. The patient should understand that taking an anticoagulant increases risks of bleeding and that the health care practitioners (HCPs) would then feel some moral blame. GPs and specialists too cannot exactly know who might suffer, though we have some risk calculators. Mrs X required reassurance from her GP that she would not suffer in future health care because of exerting informed choice. In this case, she decided to restart anticoagulation but understood that she could change her mind at any time.

Scenario: Truth telling

Mr Y attends alone to talk about his dad. Mr Y wants him to have a home visit as he is worried about him. He seems to be limping a lot and has not been out-doors for 3 weeks, but refuses a doctor.

Mr Y says, 'Can you just pop by, doctor, but he would be angry to know I had called you, so don't tell him?'
The GP refused with an explanation that not only did he have to find the patient in and expecting him, he would need to talk to him about his legs. The son reluctantly agreed to wait at dad's house for the lunchtime visit and dad accepted the situation. On taking off his shoes and socks, he had 6-in.-long toe nails growing in an arc into his foot and causing infection. The limp was corrected by podiatry and antibiotics satisfactorily.

Scenario: Truth telling in cancer care again

Many of us have been asked not to break bad news over terminal cancer to sufferers. However, it is difficult to visit and support a patient if they don't know why they are not recovering. The patient has no ability then to decide how much information, and what they would like to know about their cancer, impending terminal care and death. The doctor is deceitful and the patient has no autonomy.

The benefits of hiding information are that the patient may believe they are going to get better for longer and be less depressed at the thought of death. However, the patient may wonder why they are not recovering and the role of the GP becomes impossible. The benefits of telling patients as much about their cancer as they want to know, is that they have an honest open relationship with their doctor. This also allows the doctor to try to improve the patient's health according to their symptoms and to prevent unnecessary symptoms like constipation, vomiting and pain. The justice of truth telling is that all patients nearing the end of life have an opportunity to exert autonomy and let their GP know if they want full information about their illness and prognosis, or not. The patient remains in the driving seat of their illness as much as possible. This allows the patient to talk to their loved ones and friends about their illness and make any arrangements before death.

The large picture

ON FAILURES, ERRORS AND WHISTLE BLOWING

In 2011, Robert Francis QC published his report on *The Mid Staffordshire NHS Foundation Trust Public Inquiry*. This report examined the problems of a Trust which was investigated due to a high mortality rate and high number of complaints. On investigation, it was clear that some patients had died unnecessarily of neglect in hospital. The report stated that patients were left in soiled bedding for lengthy periods; some were not helped to eat if unable to manage themselves; some were not able to reach drinks and some staff showed a callous indifference to the patients. This was not every staff member but there was a culture of making do with poor standard care.

How had the leadership reacted when staff complained?

The report describes a culture of defensiveness, failure to scrutinise complaints, acceptance of poor standards and the complainants were sometimes victimised. Complainants lacked trust in their managers and were fearful of speaking up. Due to poor leadership behaviours, some HCPs lost jobs and some developed psychological problems after trying to raise concerns. Patients and their relatives fared no better. The Francis report, as it is sometimes known, made hundreds of recommendations.

The first for the organisation was to make the care of the patient their first concern.

We will not go into the outcomes here but it is clear from this section of the book that good, accountable high standard leaders need to create good processes and teams and finally, they should follow Aristotle in improvement of themselves and their systems. It can be difficult to raise concerns in an environment which is bullying and threatening but it is a duty of a student, doctor and other HCP to raise concerns, acting as a whistle blower, when they see poor care.

GPs can feel very isolated and vulnerable with bullying patients, or patients who just won't take 'no' for an answer. Some drug addicts will literally 'sit you out' to get one sleeping tablet, or become aggressive to get more codeine. It is important that the GP does not 'give in' as once we have the patient will return. In fact, the drug addict may let other drug addicts know that the GP is a 'soft touch'. Staff have overheard patients and their friends discussing prescribed medication acquisition in the practice car park with intent to abuse it! There is no benefit to giving in to poor prescribing, especially of drugs of abuse, but there are harms to the drug addict and to the GP if they prescribe inappropriately. Patient's autonomy should not be respected in this instance as there is a higher justice to society, providing society with a GP who does not encourage drug abuse and further prevention of patient harm. In this circumstance, the best way of managing the consultation is to talk in process rather than personal responsibility. Try a statement such as, 'I am very sorry but it is against our practice policy here to prescribe any drug ending in . . . pam, like diazepam'. You may create a similar statement yourself; it is a way of deflecting the patient from personal threats to the GP and works well.

ON CHANGE AND POSITIVITY

For GPs, the rapid never-ending changes, made possible by computerisation, from higher authorities and politicians, over the last 30 years has left many tired and unenthusiastic, i.e. 'burnt out.' For some, virtually any improvement suggested by NHS leaders would be met with distaste as what they require at present is time, continuity and an opportunity to practice their medicine without an eye to continuing change. Patients want continuity and stability so it is no surprise that GPs have the same ideals. General practice is not a creative speciality and GPs struggle to find time to develop ideas in a creative, innovative and fulfilling way and can feel frustrated. There are areas though in which GPs can positively innovate and create.

This may be in developing specialist interests, e.g. OOH GP care, dermatology clinics, minor surgery, etc. It may be working for the CCG to improve and integrate health care for their population. It may be by becoming a medical teacher and it may be by undertaking personal learning, e.g. a certificate or diploma in an area of interest. The Royal College of General Practitioners (RCGP) is keen to have its members involved and GPs can ask to review NICE guidance to see if it matches practice as a clinical advisor. If you strongly feel that general practice is not about a specialism then you can still apply, just tick all the speciality boxes! Be proud of being a generalist.

Patients can be negative. When hearing about the bereavements, social and health problems that some people suffer we can sympathise with their negativity at stages of their life. Motivating people can be difficult. Sometimes, people don't want a solution, they just want to tell the GP, and they want support. At other times though, patients may need motivating. After hearing about their problems it can be useful to ask them how they feel they can get out of their difficult situation. Patients are much more likely to have insight into the key for change for themselves than a standardised response from their GP. We can provide literature, care pathways or personal support for them and sometimes we need to offer choices about change if they don't have any. Initially though the patient must decide that they want to change behaviour but it may be that there are positive, e.g. socialisation, aspects to their unhealthy behaviour that their GPs don't understand. Having thought about stopping a behaviour, e.g. drinking alcohol, patients need a plasticity of thinking, a creative space in which to work out how they will stop and what they will do instead and enjoy. So, changing behaviour is not always about giving something up, it might be about taking up an alternative healthier behaviour.

Scenario: Stopped smoking
Mrs X had smoked heavily for years and had mild chronic obstructive pulmonary disease (COPD) at 45 years old. She had been asked to stop numerous times

*and seen the 'stop smoking clinic' on four different occasions but never stayed off
cigarettes for long after therapy. She attended one day with a cough and told the
GP she had stopped smoking.*
*GP: Why have you stopped on this occasion? I am interested to understand what
helped you.*
Patient: I don't know doctor, I just woke up one morning and decided to stop!

Change is a bit like learning. It requires us to identify that we have something
to change or to learn and to feel motivated to do it. In the above example, there
was no need to substitute a different behaviour. Decisions not to change may be
because our current knowledge and habits are meeting our needs well enough
and we are not motivated to alter. This is as true for GPs as for patients. We may
have difficulty acting in a new way. For example, GPs who have learned facts by
rote may have difficulty creatively exploring alternative diagnoses, in the same
way that an alcoholic may always reach for a drink of whisky if upset. They may
offer the same solution to a presentation constantly and have difficulty changing
behaviour when that treatment is not effective or no longer best practice. The
secret to motivation, positivity and changing behaviour is nurturing an area of
thinking which is creative and wants to investigate new ideas. Exploring new
ideas keeps us bright, whether we are patients, GPs or both. In changing behaviour patients and doctors may relapse and should re-explore their motivation and
changes before retrying and succeeding.

APPRENTICESHIP–MASTER MODEL OF MEDICAL EDUCATION

Medical students train for 4–6 years at university and spend most of their clinical undergraduate course years in hospitals and GP practices. Here they meet
patients and develop their knowledge, skills and behaviours to qualify as doctors. In hospitals and GP practices, they meet medical teams with primary and
secondary care specialists. Students in general practice have close contact with
their primary care specialists. They may see patients on their own, sit in with GP
clinics or with other members of the primary care team, depending on the
requirements of the students and the module. Even if the student is to see patients
alone and then report back most GPs will sit their student in with them initially
to check their standards, professionalism and competency for their level. The GP
can then decide the student's fitness to see patients that the GP is responsible for.
Doctors training in Foundation posts and GP speciality trainees also train in GP
practices. GP tutors (in postgraduate training also called GP trainers), assess the
competency of their learners, related to their stage of training. The various
learners will therefore watch their GP trainer and perceive them as role models.
This is known to be an important learning and teaching strategy. GP teaching
involves acting as expert and master in an apprentice-master relationship.
Learners model themselves on the behaviours they see. Ethically, trainers must
offer high professional and personal standards, continually to provide good role
modelling.

Scenario: Negative role modelling

Medical student: 'I want to let you know that my student partner is upset. When the GP asked him a question, he told me that the GP was abrupt and rude and said, "That's wrong, you won't qualify"'.

The effect of this was that both students felt unable to answer questions from this GP as they didn't want to be humiliated.

Scenario: Negative role modelling

GP Registrar: 'My GP trainer keeps the clinic room very cold and says it is so the patients won't stay as long!'

Scenario: Positive role modelling

Student: 'I love my general practice placement. The GP is so enthusiastic and encouraging. He gives me time to discuss cases and asks questions. The patients are lovely. I have been to diabetic clinic and baby clinic too and the nurses knew what I needed to learn and were so helpful'.

In 1956, Bloom developed a taxonomy of learning in which recall of facts was at the lowest level and higher levels of learning involved thinking and reasoning. Higher levels of learning may not be more important than knowing some facts but by building on successive layers of learning the doctor reaches expertise. Using high levels of learning in general practice might happen when setting up new care pathways or writing new guidance. This taxonomy was later revised by Krathwol in 2000* and is below.

Clinical learners enter the GP practice at the 'applying' stage having learned important facts and understood them.

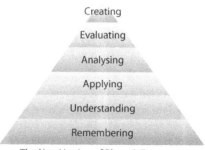

The New Version of Bloom's Taxonomy

(From https://www.flickr.com/photos/21847073@N05/5857112597)

---

* Krathwohl DR. A revision of Bloom's taxonomy: An overview. *Theory Into Practice* 2002; 41(4):212–218.

At this stage, the master-apprenticeship model requires GP tutors to acquire teaching skills layered on top of their consultation skills to use within the consultations for both the patient and the learner. These are

- Knowledge
- Skills: medical and teaching
- Behaviours: professionalism, enthusiasm and commitment
- Time and clarity of teaching outcomes

The last requirement of time and process can be difficult within the usual working day and organisations employing GP tutors need to help facilitate this. The diagram below incorporates the GP tutor-apprentice learning and teaching which may also occur within our GP consultations:

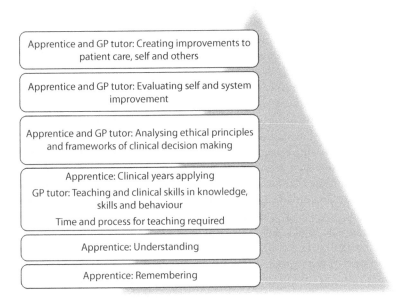

How we learn on the job: Teams and leaders

GPs act as leaders and team workers throughout their career to improve patient care. They are part of the primary care team and work in teams with patients and their families at times. Optimising these skills benefits the patient and consultation so is discussed in this consultation section.

Trainer: Give me an example of team working.
Trainee: Sure. I met a patient with a leg ulcer and referred them to the district nurses for management.
Trainer: That's not team work. That's called making a referral.

Teams were trendy, with lots of emphasis on the primary care team in GP publications and postgraduate education for a couple of decades. Now 'leadership' is the buzzword. Whole buildings and policies are currently invested in the development of medical leaders and streaming early career stage clinicians into leadership roles. It is a possibility that experienced full-time clinicians or late developers might be disadvantaged by early career pathways and young career leaders may not fully understand the roles they will lead if never full-time for a significant part of their careers. For GP partners to run practices, employ staff, offer high standard health services to patients and maintain their knowledge bases, GPs must variously act as leaders, managers and team players. Training helps in all these roles. The movement of large swathes of GPs into clinical commissioning groups (CCGs) and wider NHS bodies also requires leadership and team-building training and some organisations do this, others do not.

TEAMS

Teams require a leader. The leadership skill required is accurate skill identification with distribution of those skills to the correct individuals and oversight of process and progress. Team members should own their roles and understand them as a part of the whole team, leading on their responsibilities. Members should be able to run effortlessly, depending on their interest and need, between leadership and team roles. It is unfortunate that the term 'leader' is associated with higher repute than 'team worker', when both are invaluable and roles should be fluid over different tasks.

Teams ebb and flow and a stable team requires trust between its members, knowing that everyone is committed and able to do their job to achieve an excellent output. Teams do not have a life span if there are still goals to achieve but a team may come together for a specific task (or all tasks are completed) and then disbands. In general practice, tasks are never all completed so the teams we work with are enduring, trusting and interesting.

Tuckman described a developmental model of group formation comprising: forming, storming, norming and performing. This is summarised below to give GPs oversight of some group dynamics when entering new teams.

Forming: This starting phase orientates around members testing normal behaviours for the group. This is discovering the behaviours between individuals and boundaries of the task. At this stage members are dependent largely on the leader, other group members and pre-existing standards which have been imported into the group. Group members therefore uncover the 'ground rules' in personal and task related areas.

Storming: This is the stage in which the group may exhibit emotion, resistance and conflict. At this stage group members may test out their abilities to change the ground rules uncovered in forming, they may bring existing emotions into the group and they may have strong emotions about other group members or the task in hand.

Norming: Here the group pulls together, new standards are adopted and new roles evolve. Personal opinions can be expressed and positive group relationships are developed.

Performing: This group is functional and focuses on the task. Members understand their roles, which are flexible and functional. The ground rules, the underlying structure or processes are supportive of the task. The team is strategically aware and able to work well to complete the tasks.

The speed at which a new group runs through the stages varies and depends on the personalities and personal dependency of its members. In the forming section, the leadership role is important in providing information about the task, roles, ground rules, i.e. expected norms of behaviour and actions. By the performing stage, the role of the leader is reduced and can be very flexible. The leader may provide overseer function and other members may take up leadership roles at times. A leader may not be required for large amounts of performance. When groups finish, unlikely in GP but common on committees brought together for shorter term outcomes, there can be a sense of loss. Individuals may miss hearing and relating to some excellent individuals when tasks have been completed and the committee disbanded. Being aware of these processes helps us mature as group members and leaders.

There has been much written about roles of group members and we are not going to discuss all this here, largely because there are very many descriptions and some of them are restrictive, fragmenting individual talents which may, if nurtured, roam over roles. Nevertheless, some group members are more instigators than others; some more likely to be given a set task and do it well; some more likely to have an eye to process and outcomes and keep the group on track over performance and time; some are more strategic thinkers and problem solvers in a way that other members aren't. Some team members are enthusiasts and motivate the group. Some may interrupt and over-talk members and others are quiet and will contribute only if directly asked. As GPs, we should bring our skills with a generosity of spirit or not join the group at all. This may mean turning down opportunities and there can be anxiety, especially at early career stages, that the opportunity won't return. If you are curious intellectually, high standard and create time to join a group and help with the outcomes you will always be offered more opportunities over time.

In setting up a group ask the following questions:

- What is this team going to achieve?
- Are the members the best choice for the task?
- Has selection been fair?
- Is there time allocated for this group to perform?
- Is there a leader/facilitator?
- Is there someone to take minutes, distribute agreed action plans and arrange rooms, etc.?
- Is the group process clear?
- Is the group improving and are members given an opportunity to improve transferable skills, emotionally and physically related to the task?
- Is there space for members to discuss, improve and create change if required?
- How will the group know if it has achieved success? How will success be measured?

Primary care team formation may be initially difficult due to hierarchies amongst GPs and other HCPs. In setting up a group, it is important that the background experience of the individuals is thought through and they are given confidence to contribute. The GP may lead on clinical governance and create guidelines for the practice. Nowadays though, many of these are 'off the peg' from expert bodies. Guideline writing is partly person specific in style and involves the main user, perhaps this is the assistant practitioner (AP), to act as lead author to create the next guideline may make them more usable. The GP should remain an involved group member. Delegating doesn't mean leaving the group because 'there is something more pressing to do', it means working closely with nursing and health assistants (HA) as colleagues. So, a guideline on cholesterol management written by an AP may be more useable to the practice than one written by the GP and bring GPs, nurses and APs together intellectually, following national protocols but fitting all the various patient groups and upskilling practice team members. These activities also create some fun, lasting friendship and trust. Patient members can be incorporated onto these teams and can sometimes shed light on the personal reasons which prevent guidelines from working but which are not immediately obvious to medical staff. Patients may have helpful views on the patient onus of clinic visits, tablets, wanted information about common side effects of medications and so on.

The reality of extended primary care teams is that GPs are not usually a part of their team: there are several different professionals to whom we refer, usually by e-mail; the community drug team, social work team, health visitors, physiotherapists and even the district nurses. These are not individuals we meet daily and share experiences closely with. They are referred to and communicated with but are often not teams in a truly productive sense.

So, who is the main team in the practice?

This should be our practice partners and other HCPs, including the practice receptionists but again, this requires regular space for team formation and discussion. Some practices do meet meaningfully but many are inundated with work and have no time to meet in the true spirit of team work. GPs can spend all day in clinics and visits and not meet another doctor. This isolation can lead to problems if difficulties arise, as the doctor may forget, or not be aware that other HCPs on the premises could help him/her out.

Scenario: Where are our colleagues?
A GP sat at her desk sweating and upset with the workload. It was hot and she had just seen 18 patients and completed six phone consultations. The computer messaged that she had three visits before afternoon surgery. I had popped over with a cremation form request and noticed that her hands were shaking and her shirt drenched with sweat. On asking her, there were three other GPs and two practice nurses in the building, but she hadn't asked them for help because she was too busy and not aware of them as a part of her team. I suggested that she phone them for help and that we would leave my request for another time.

Similar scenarios have been related; some GPs have burst into tears, some pace about and some retire early or take long-term sickness as they have not been supported by their practice teams. It might not be the team's fault if they did not know the issues, but if asked for help, they should offer it. It is a sign of the times that many colleagues, when discussing this, feel their own workloads are so high, they are sometimes unhelpful in response over workloads. This stress leads to doctors working when ill, e.g. one GP used to vomit with severe migraine between patients but carry on afterwards.

The main team in the practice which usually runs with excellence is the team in the clinic room: GP and patient, and their carer if present. Without the formation of trust and unity to a common purpose of health improvement, our consultations are meaningless. GPs facilitate patients and their carers to improve health and within that short consultation enduring teams are formed.

LEADERS: COPS, ROBBERS AND MAGISTRATES

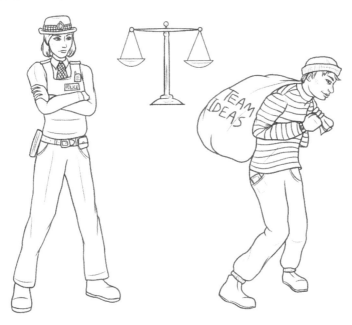

Cops, robbers and magistrates.

There are lots of ways to become an effective leader. GPs may choose to lead by example; they may lead from the back seat, encouraging and training team members to achieve outcomes or may choose to lead by authority. Better still, we may develop leadership skills so that we move between these skills, depending on the problem. Good leaders create good teams and outcomes. Some, however, don't develop the middle ground of skills and act only as cops, or robbers!

Being a cop: There is no point leading by training and consensus when a patient attends with an acute myocardial infarction. The priority is to lead with authority to attain a quick positive resolution for your patient. This is like being a good cop; applying the law (clinical guidelines and good clinical practice) quickly and successfully so that the patient doesn't suffer. Afterwards though, there may be a training requirement or discussion with members about what they saw and felt, especially if someone has died or been part of a violent act, like a road accident. Blaming a colleague for not being quick enough with the defibrillator doesn't help. In fact, good leaders are experts at predicting consequences of their actions and there is no long-term positive outcome to apportioning guilt and anxiety. Discussing care and how to improve to achieve best care next time requires skilled leadership.

Cops may be excellent in emergency scenarios but there are also bad cops. Leadership by dogmatism and bullying does not create good team work or attract motivated team members. Sarcasm, shouting or blaming have no place in leadership skills yet are encountered in organisations. Indeed, *The Shipman report* of 2005, by Dame Janet Smith wrote that Dr Harold Shipman, a much-loved local GP, who was convicted of murdering 15 patients and almost certainly killing 250 or more, ran a single-handed practice in which staff did not feel able to challenge his actions. His practice nurse deferred to him and felt unable to question him over deaths in practice, even though there is an example of Dr Shipman attempting resuscitation with her on a patient he had killed. In this case, the emergency trolley was not brought to the patient or used. Ironically, he was a murderer acting in this leadership model as a cop but as a bad cop. Harold Shipman could dominate his staff as a bully.

Emergencies may not always be well handled but team working to improve processes is described below.

Scenario: Primary care emergency

Mr Y is 52 years old and a diabetic. He develops slurred speech in a nearby café whilst out with his wife. She drives him to the health centre and runs in to ask for help. The receptionist calls the GP who attends the patient in the carpark as Mr Y is too unwell to get out of the car. The GP turns around to ask the receptionist for a capillary blood glucose monitor and a 999 call, to find he is on his own.

Following this, the index practice met and wrote a protocol stating that two staff members, the emergency kit and two doctors should attend an emergency initially and the lead GP should stand individuals down when satisfied he or she didn't need more help. The practice improvement activity was recorded in team members' appraisals. The next time an emergency arose, it was due to a patient with anaphylaxis. To be precise, Miss X had urticaria, lip swelling, acute wheezing and breathlessness. The practice's emergency care was exceptionally well organised, the GP felt supported by colleagues and the team could practice their skills. GPs don't see many emergencies, so combined thinking and skills is also helpful rather than acting alone.

Unlike Harold Shipman, GPs are not murderers, they are caring doctors but if stressed and unable to cope, they may develop unhelpful leadership styles such as anger, sarcasm and bullying and become bad cops.

Being a robber: These are leaders who take personal credit for other team members' work to improve their own status, without recognising or developing the team. The good leader is explicit with team members about where credit lies and how that will be publicised if appropriate. If team members at any level of employment are not valued, heard or developed they will lose interest, become resentful and may become destructive in meetings. Mostly though, they keep their heads down and do what they are told. This enables protocols and processes to work satisfactorily but without improvement, and without improvement for self or patients there is little motivation.

Being a magistrate: (derivation: *magister* in Latin meaning master.) The ancient Romans had magistrates who upheld the law.

There are at least five aspects to a successful leader acting here as a magistrate:

1. Understanding the task and team requirements and creating effective processes to achieve them
2. Identifying successes or problems early, so retaining an overarching view and taking overall responsibility, whilst delegating task responsibilities
3. Developing team members in both tasks and development, including encouraging a sense of fulfilment or fun when possible
4. Self-improvement in the leaders' leadership and team work
5. Knowing when teams no longer require leadership; the leader can then enjoy being a full team member in a high-performance team

The NHS has a leadership academy and I would urge GPs and HCPs to explore their model and think about how it might relate to our own work and role.

Useful Resources:

- An interesting site if you would like to explore more about medical ethics: *UKCEN Clinical Ethics Network at* http://www.ukcen.net/ethical_issues /ethical_frameworks/the_four_principles_of_biomedical_ethics
- Bruce W. Tuckman – forming, storming norming and performing in groups from infed http://infed.org/mobi/bruce-w-tuckman-forming-storming-norming-and-performing-in-groups/
- Healthcare Leadership Model: the NHS Leadership Academy at www. leadershipacademy.nhs.uk
- Further reading on the Shipman reports at: http://webarchive.nationalarchives. gov.uk/20090808154959/http://www.the-shipman-inquiry.org.uk/5r_page. asp?ID=4565

Gifts

We all want to be appreciated and thanked but a card is worth more than a present. Honestly, there are ethical aspects to accepting gifts from patients, though they are commonly offered. Presents are problematic. Any gift over £100 must be listed on a register with the name of the donor, NHS number or address, nature of gift and estimated value. The GMC advises GPs not to encourage patients to gift, lend or bequeath anything to them. GPs are allowed to accept unsolicited gifts, so long as it does not affect the patient–doctor relationship and actions in any way. In fact, refusing a gift can seem very rude at times. Gifts and cards should be kept for appraisal discussions; it is nice to review them and know that your work has been appreciated. For every one person who has gone to the trouble to write to the GP, there are lots more who are singing their praises which they don't hear. A GP related that her mother flew back from a holiday and sat next to a patient who said what a wonderful GP she had – only to find it was her husband! She never heard the end of it, mother-in-law was so proud!

Best presents I have received are: a cabbage which was left over from the allotment; rhubarb; a bag of buy-one-get-one free potatoes which the patient wondered if the GP would like as she only needed one; poems; £20 as part of a bingo win.

I refused the £20 and the elderly lady said she was walking out and leaving it on the desk. I wondered what to do with the £20 and bought a National Geographic subscription to enjoy and then put them in the waiting area after for patients to browse. Flowers of course.

Then there was the man who always gave his GP half a packet of polo mints. The GP tried to keep to time to see if she could ever get the full packet (was he starting on them in the waiting area?) but no, always half a packet.

Most presents though do come, however inadvertently by the patient, with a feeling that the GP should be available to see that patient personally and in that sense, there can be a feeling of being morally bought.

To avoid this, suggesting to the present giver that all the staff share in the chocolates or biscuits can make it less personal and shares the luck with other staff too. A patient told his GP that he would bring in a dozen loaves as a thank-you one day. The GP didn't think he had done much medically evidently. Anyway, the GP sought to head off the gift by stating that he would share them round the staff. The next week the deputy manager knocked on the clinic door with a box of loaves. The GP suggested the staff member share them round the staff and the GP take one. The deputy manager responded that two boxes had arrived, one for the staff and one box for the GP! A few patients went home with loaves that day too! How generous, and a lot of fun and smiles all round! Another GP was given a bicycle and felt obligated to refuse. Unfortunately, the donor became quite upset and left it with the GP despite her protests. The GP that evening felt so uncomfortable that she took the bike round to the patient's house and returned it but was left feeling that she had caused a lot of upset. Basically, the monetary value had crossed a line for this GP and we all must decide our own value and keep it low in monetary terms.

Removing patients

It is a shame when patients we have known for years move away, and some even check whether they can keep their GP before deciding where to move! Patients can be removed if they have moved out of the practice area, but with a 30-day limit to find another GP before removal. However, there may be a breakdown of the doctor–patient relationship and for reasons of violence, stealing, verbal, physical, sexual, racial abuse or other unreasonable behaviour the practice may wish to remove a patient from the list. The patient should be told, if possible in writing and first with a warning letter, unless the removal is due to a change of address or would be harmful to the physical or mental health of the patient or there is a risk to the safety of staff, the practice, visitors or it is just not possible to do so. Retain the explanation for removal for National Health Service England (NHSE). Once removing the patient, the practice informs NHSE in writing and the removal takes place after the eighth day of the request being received by NHSE.

If a patient is violent and the police have been involved or informed, removal can be immediate if the GP, HCP or other practice staff feel threatened. Complaints against the practice though are not a reason to remove a patient unless there are other reasons to suggest a relationship breakdown between doctor and patient, such as an unfounded complaint or allegation or a personal attack on members of staff. Patients can't be removed because treatments are expensive, or for particular clinical conditions, age, race, gender, social class, religion, sexual orientation or appearance. We all recognize this as discrimination and GPs do not discriminate.

Family members should not be removed because one family member, who is a patient, is removed. The exception is if visiting the home of the remaining family on the practice list would cause confrontation, especially violence.

It is easiest to have this policy clearly in the practice leaflet and website.

The GMC have clear advice on their website: http://www.gmc-uk.org/guidance/ethical_guidance/30182.asp.

Complaints

Patients have a right to complain and should not be removed from the practice because they have exercised this right. Most often, patient complaints improve care and the practice should have a clear complaints policy available to patients. Most complaints are settled by having a GP who listens and acknowledges the issue. This may not even require a complaint procedure to be formalised, some patients bring up issues in practice and are satisfied when asked if they want to pursue a complaint more formally and decline. If the practice complaints procedure is invoked, the practice manager will follow the complaint and it is the duty of the GP to respond to the complaint in a timely way. The GP should meet with the patient and with the practice manager. It might be helpful for the patient to bring a friend or relative for moral support as complaining is daunting. Offer a clear explanation and apology, if appropriate with a clear action plan on how to improve for next time. In our experience, almost everyone complaining wants an apology and acknowledgement that the care given was not the best. If complaints are not settled informally, then the patient can go on to more formal actions.

Religion and culture

In this section, I explore effects of religion and culture on both the GP and the patient. We focus on Catholicism, Judaism and Islam as religions (Catholics, Jews and Muslims) with a short discussion of specific Jehovah's Witness issues in medicine.

We know that our own moral codes are a part of our background, our experiences, our personalities and our beliefs. We also develop mental stereotypes for religious and cultural groups. Stereotypes can be helpful shortcuts to good practice but not always. They are like making immediate diagnoses due to pattern recognition. For instance, a GP may instantly recognise a basal cell cancer (BCC) on an older person's skin because it has a pearly edge, associated telangiectasia and central scabbed-over crater. However, if pattern recognition lets the clinician down, e.g. it is not a BCC, it is an absolute mistake; a definite mistaken diagnosis which might be difficult to shake off mentally.

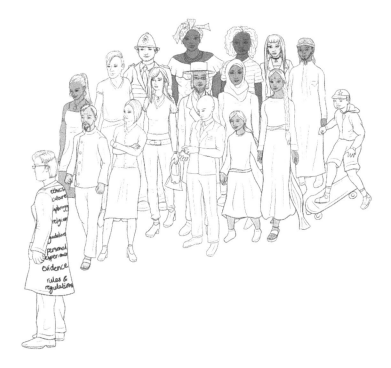

We may bring religion, beliefs and cultures to consultations.

Scenario: Incorrect pattern recognition of pain

Mrs X, 58 years old, attends her GP with left-sided thigh pain. She is a nurse so moves patients about and thinks this is the cause. There are no other symptoms and no signs. She has good back and hip movements and is diagnosed with a left quadriceps sprain and referred to physiotherapy. The physiotherapist agrees with the diagnosis but treatment and time didn't help. Mrs X continued to complain of pain and took several medications for it and was eventually referred by to the local musculoskeletal clinic. Ten months later, she was diagnosed with a prolapsed intervertebral disc and offered surgery. The pain went away after surgery.

In this case, the initial diagnosis of quadriceps sprain fitted everyone's diagnostic pattern and it was some time before the true cause, in a woman with no back pain and excellent back movements, could be diagnosed.

In the same way, the line between stereotypy (assuming a truth) and discrimination (that the truth may not hold for the person before you) is a fine one. A typical expectation would be to assume that Muslim or Jewish women would only see a female clinician. Many patients, regardless of culture or religion, will prefer to see the clinician that they believe will do them the most good, is knowledgeable and interested in helping them, before deciding on sex preferences. People do make decisions based on their culture, family experiences and their religion but these may vary between individuals and over time and their own patient context. Living in a liberal UK society may lead to varying interpretations of beliefs and clinicians should recognise religious and cultural preferences but be aware that they are not a truism for all peoples. One of the best ways of connecting, and not offending people of different cultures from our own, is to ask them if there are things they are anxious about or might be offended by. Say to the patient, 'If I am suggesting something you find culturally difficult or rude it is not intentional so please let me know'.

An Asian GP related feeling anxious when meeting a white patient who was covered in Nazi tattoos and racist comments, but who actually conducted himself in an extremely pleasant manner. People can change and aren't always as we prejudge them to be.

Religious people vary in their religiosity too, so there are orthodox and liberal views of religions. We will use the term 'strict' to describe the more traditional orthodox views but of course, many people are 'strict' about a more liberal version of their religion. The wording is for clarity, not to offend.

Islam is divided into different forms; two of which are Shia and Sunni so there may be differing interpretations within Islam.

Catholics and Protestants may have different views, e.g. over contraception but some Catholics use birth control whilst more strictly interpretive Catholics don't, but they are all Christians.

Finally, not everyone from a religious background has to be religious themselves. People may also pick which parts of their religion they believe to be important. As one patient said to me, *'I am gay. Gay Muslim men may come to countries where they can live their lives without fear'.*

It can be interesting and useful though to have some idea of issues which may affect those who hold religious beliefs. Below is a short synopsis of some visible symbols and religious customs of interest to the reader. Although of general interest, I hope some of the facts allow GPs to be sensitive to cultural and religious diversity.

One recent problem for instance, has been the realisation that pork gelatine may be found in some medication capsules, including vitamin D. People who cover up due to cultural or religious beliefs are more prone to vitamin D deficiency as 90% of vitamin D is made through the action of sunlight on our skins. Low vitamin D leads to osteomalacia, but some of these people will not consume pork- or beef-based medications as treatment. Being aware of this allows the GP to provide acceptable alternatives and improve treatment compliance.

Young people, or indeed anyone, may rebel against their cultural or religious beliefs or lose belief. It may be that in those circumstances and if in trouble, e.g. a young girl belonging to any group that does not allow sex before marriage or abortion, who finds herself with an unexpected pregnancy, may avoid a doctor of the same background faith, in order to avoid censure.

Some cultural groups have an 'honour-'based system which defines the roles of men and women within their culture. This may lead to conflicts within families, which GPs may have considered close and non-abusive, as young people adapt to living in a Western secular society. An example would be a young woman not wanting an arranged marriage within or outside the United Kingdom. This is illegal in the United Kingdom and clinicians may become aware of tensions and need to protect the victim.*

EXPLORING JEHOVAH'S WITNESSES, CATHOLICISM, JUDAISM AND ISLAM

Jehovah's witnesses

Jehovah's witnesses avoid blood transfusions and over years, they have given impetus to blood transfusion substitutes and bloodless surgery. They may carry an Advance Decision to Refuse Treatment (ADRT) document which states which blood products are and are not acceptable. Usually whole blood transfusion is not acceptable but clotting factors, albumen and immunoglobulin derivatives may be acceptable.†

---

* This site contains contact details for GPs concerned that a patient is being forced against their will to marry. There is a different contact detail in Scotland: Forced Marriage https://www.gov.uk/stop-forced-marriage.

† Joint United Kingdom (UK) Blood Transfusion and Tissue Transplantation Services Professional Advisory Committee at: http://www.transfusionguidelines.org/transfusion -handbook/12-management-of-patients-who-do-not-accept-transfusion/12-2-jehovah -s-witnesses-and-blood-transfusion.

Catholicism

Catholicism is led by the Pope who resides in Rome and is the living will of Saint Peter, a disciple of Jesus who is considered the son of God. All priests are men. Strict Catholic adherence prohibits abstinence of sex and use of contraceptives, other than natural family planning. Natural family planning means timing sexual intercourse to take advantage of the least fertile stages of the woman's menstrual cycle. Abortion is considered a sin to strict Catholics and the Abortion Act does not cover Northern Ireland, where other laws are used to allow abortion in more serious threats to maternal health than in the rest of the United Kingdom. That is, that there must be serious permanent, physical or mental ill health to the mother if the pregnancy is continued.

Strict Catholics may not eat meat on Fridays (fish is permissible) and they may fast, which means one meal a day, on Ash Wednesday and Good Friday. In addition, they may fast for 1 hour before mass. This applies to those aged 18–60 years but anyone with illness is exempted.*

Catholic priests give prayers for the sick to the patient at the end of life and patients are more likely to be buried, but cremation can be allowed.

Judaism

Jews believe in one God and follow laws and texts written in the Torah. Their religious leader is the rabbi. Jews recite prayers three times a day and Jewish men may be obvious to non-Jews because they wear a skull cap (kippah). Some strict orthodox Jews wear overcoats, hats, hair of ringlets and prayer shawls with tassels.

Strict Jews take the 8-day Passover week off as holiday and their Shabbat starts at sunset on Fridays to nightfall on Saturdays. So, Jewish colleagues may request on Fridays early finishes from work, and Jewish patients may not want to attend their GP then. During Shabbat, Jews should not work and should not drive their cars. This accounts for some Jewish communities living close to synagogues. The most Holy days, associated with synagogue attendance, prayer and fasting are Yom Kippur and Rosh Hashanah. Jewish homes have a small enclosed script affixed to the doorway of their homes and sometimes of work, like the GP clinic doorway, the Mezuzah.

Jews are forbidden from eating shellfish and pork. Foods which are allowed are termed Kosher. Pork products include gelatine and once, when offering marshmallows and other gummy sweets round students, Jewish and Muslim students pointed out that unfortunately, gelatin was forbidden and they would abstain from the sweets.

For strict Jews, a woman menstruating should not have sex until 7 days after the end of her period. Men may sleep in a separate bed when their wife is menstruating. This may have repercussions for women wanting to conceive. Strict Jewish orders do not allow contraception and male sterilisation is forbidden but

---

* https://www.ewtn.com/faith/lent/fast.htm

more liberal groups do allow contraceptive use, according to individual conscience. Jewish boys are circumcised on day 8 of life and so have no foreskin.

Some strict Jewish groups segregate men and women at all times, and would not be comfortable exchanging a handshake or a hug with a person of the opposite sex.

On death, synagogue members usually prepare bodies for burial and there is 7 days of mourning, in which the bereaved relative is house-bound. The dead body is washed and wrapped in a sheet and strict Jewish men are buried in their prayer shawls. Cremation and embalming are forbidden to strict Jews but may be allowed in the more liberal groups. Burial occurs as soon as possible after death and is in Jewish cemeteries.

Islam

Muslims follow Islam, they believe in one God, called Allah, and follow the teaching written in the Quran (Koran) and the prophet Muhammad. Their religious leaders are imams and are men. Islamic customs vary over many different countries.

On birth, a Muslim elder may say a prayer to the infant shortly after birth. Usually Muslim men are circumcised. Muslim doctors may receive requests for private referrals for circumcisions on religious grounds. This can be done at any age but is usually performed in early infancy. Some Muslim predominant cultures abroad allow female genital mutilation (FGM) but this is not a religious custom and is illegal in the United Kingdom.

Prayers are said five times a day facing Mecca and after ritual washing of hands, face and feet. Where water is not available, this can be done symbolically. For Muslims with incontinence issues this can have a profound psychological effect as they may not feel clean for prayer. The prayers are short and tend not to interfere with the running of the day as a Muslim GP. Communal formal prayers are on Friday, in the early afternoon, but there is no ostracisation for non-attendance.

Adult Muslims observe a month of fasting during daylight hours, ending with a celebration, Eid. Although there is a more philosophical purpose to Ramadan, it means Muslims may fast from food and water and restrain from sex during dawn to dusk. There are exemptions for fasting for nursing mothers, menstruating women whilst on their period, ill people, e.g. diabetics. However, we have experienced diabetic elderly Muslims who, despite knowing they could be exempt from fasting in Ramadan, do fast and this has implications for blood pressure and diabetic treatments. Ramadan follows a lunar calendar so the dates have a 36-year cycle. In winter, the day is short but long 16-hour days of fasting in the summer can be difficult for some people. Strict Muslims may include fasting from tablets and injections, so this should be discussed with the patients as usual treatment regimens may not be adhered to. It is an ambition of religious Muslims to go on pilgrimage, and occasionally receiving postcards from patients on pilgrimage is very interesting. Generally, patients will want the meningitis ACWY vaccination as a requirement to enter Saudi Arabia on pilgrimage. As meningitis W increased in incidence, the Joint Committee on Vaccination and Immunisation (JCVI) introduced routine quadrivalent meningitis ACWY vaccination to 18-year olds in 2016, so some young patients will have been vaccinated.*

Muslims do not eat pork and its products, including bacon and ham and do not eat pork gelatine. Some do not eat beef gelatine either. Their food, if strict Muslims, should be Halal prepared. Kosher prepared food is also acceptable to Muslims. Strict Muslims are teetotal, including alcohol in mouth washes, etc.

Men and women are equal but there is a traditional view that men are earners and women stay at home with the children. There are sometimes tensions requiring women to treat children and females and male GPs to treat men in Muslim countries, which are obviously not followed in the United Kingdom. But Muslims may ask for gender preferences in their GPs if possible. Muslim women who are strict may find it difficult to expose their arms as doctors (for washing, in theatre, etc.) and they often wear a head scarf (hijab) covering the head but not the face so that they can communicate clearly with their patients. Some Muslim women patients however are completely covered, except for their eyes and the Islamic faith supports modesty in covering up. Devout Muslim men will usually cover up to their knees and some Muslim men wear head caps. As a part of modesty, Muslims may not offer direct eye contact easily with the opposite sex, this is at variance with the Western habit of conversation. They will not welcome handshakes or other physical contact with members of the opposite sex. The problem for examination is most likely to occur in intimate examinations. Some years ago, a Muslim patient came with her husband to see a GP and refused to uncover her chest for auscultation adequately. She had attended with a dry cough and the consultation was via an interpreter. She did not appear breathless and seemed fairly well. He arranged a chest x-ray due to inability to properly auscultate the chest, which revealed a large pleural effusion due to tuberculosis.

Muslims do not usually agree with abortion except in cases of severe risk to maternal life and do not agree with sterilisation. Some Muslims believe that the soul enters the fetal body at 120 days of existence (16 weeks gestation) so terminations may be less acceptable after that time.

At death, Muslims are washed and shrouded by volunteers from the Mosque and buried facing Mecca. Muslims usually mourn for a month but widows for 4 months. In the first 3 days after death, the community feed the bereaved family members. Post mortems are not usually wanted by Muslims so coroners may offer magnetic resonance imaging (MRI) scanning to families where causes of death are unknown. Cremation is generally forbidden.

Finally, a note that many Hindus will avoid beef and some will be vegetarian. Patients entering pregnancy who are vegetarian, Hindu or not, have sometimes been severely anaemic at onset with iron and vitamin B_{12} deficiency.

So, keep an open mind, each person is an individual and awareness and communication are important.

* Enhanced Service Specification Meningococcal ACWY (MenACWY) 18 years on 31 August vaccination programme 2016/17 at: https://www.england.nhs.uk/commission ing/wp-content/uploads/sites/12/2016/04/MenACWY-2016-17.pdf.

Interpreters

Most GPs have patients for whom English is not their first language. Indeed an 80-year-old lady related that when she was first in the United Kingdom as a young woman, she was driven by her husband each Sunday 60 miles to the nearest family who spoke her language. The rest of the week there was just her husband to speak to! It is difficult to imagine that sort of isolation. Ask patients which language they prefer to speak in and make a note in their records. Sometimes, young children or spouses with excellent English come into the clinic as the interpreter; the husband usually for his wife. This is not acceptable although occasionally the patient insists and shows the doctor something minor, like an eczema and the consultation goes ahead. This is less than good practice though. More likely, there is something personal – symptoms of a urinary tract infection, period problems, contraception requests, mental health concerns and these require a professional interpreting service to prevent bias and promote patient understanding and autonomy.

Scenario: Why family interpreters can be a problem
A young couple attend their GP.

Mr Y: My wife has pain on passing urine.
GP: Thank you for bringing her. Does she not have much English?
Mr Y: Hardly any.
GP: What language does she speak? I would like to phone up an interpreter for her and you can then wait outside for her.
Mr Y: No. no, I am a good interpreter, I have come specially to help (repeated despite GP protestations).
GP: Okay, but you must ask her exactly what I say and repeat exactly back to me what she answers, is that okay?
Mr Y: Yes of course, doctor.
GP: (asks about symptoms of urinary tract infection and then asks) Do you have regular periods?
Mr Y: (looks embarrassed and says) 'Yes she does' (without asking her).
GP: No, you must interpret and ask her (Mr Y does reluctantly).
GP: Is there any chance you could be pregnant?
Mr Y: No! (again, he does not ask her before replying).
GP: Can you ask her please? I think we do need an interpreter used to women's health problems. I will phone up the interpreter line and you can relax outside for a few minutes.

Mr Y fled! At the end of the phone conversation, in which this quiet, embarrassed woman became animated and witty and the GP gained a small insight into her personality, it was important to establish permission about what information the GP was to pass on to the husband.

The interpreting service can be booked and an interpreter can accompany the patient. This provides a friendly face and sometimes continuity. Alternatively, there is an interpreter language telephone line which is amazingly quick at finding any language, even ones you have never heard of. As confidentiality can be a burden, having an interpreter on the end of a phone, who does not know or see the patient may be helpful.

For instance, a GP attended a community centre to talk to a group of middle-aged and older women of Asian origin about women's health. The interpreter giggled and looked embarrassed when the word sex was used and refused to interpret. It was clear some of the women knew what the conversation was about and a few passed on the interpretation and a giggle went around. On discussing risks of cervical cancer and sexually transmitted infections (STIs), the official interpreter was too embarrassed to continue and would not interpret the words 'sex outside of marriage'. Again, a few other heads spread the news round. At the end, the group were asked if anything had been missed out and a few older women said it had been very interesting but they had wanted to talk about depression and loneliness.

Conscientious objection to abortion and to contraception

Sometimes, there is a conflict between personal and professional ethical values. In important areas, ethics are debated by society's leaders and placed into laws and regulations and the GMC website is an excellent resource for GPs. Many doctors will have religious or personal views for and against abortion, especially when the reasons for abortion are due to adverse social circumstances rather than adverse physical health problems. In these circumstances, doctors who conscientiously object to abortion may refuse to refer patients for the procedure. However, the GMC makes it clear that the doctor concerned must offer the patient an alternative GP who will manage the patient's request. In ethical terms, this means that the doctor is no longer directly responsible for the medical preparation of the abortion. For some GPs though, passing the case to another to facilitate the abortion may not feel like innocence. The same rule applies to provision of contraception or any other procedure. GPs must never discriminate against patients due to their own beliefs or offer their own beliefs to their patients to cause them distress. Patients are vulnerable when making decisions about their care and require impartial medical advice, working in the best interests of that patient at that time. Where views differ between GPs and patients the GP may feel they want to disclose the issue to another but it is very important to retain patient confidentiality. GPs should ensure the practice is aware of any conscientious objections they have and this information should be available in the practice leaflet, a poster in the practice and online at the practice website for patients to view. Hopefully, patients might be able to select the GP that will be able to offer them appropriate care.

Useful Resources:

- GMC advice on personal beliefs and medical practice at: http://www.gmc-uk .org/static/documents/content/Personal_beliefs-web.pdf.Ethics and behaviours 141

Appraisal and revalidation

This short section highlights appraisals and revalidation. In the consultation, doctors uncover areas of practice and knowledge that they want to improve or describe as part of their appraisal. They may want to act upon a valid complaint or analyse a good clinical diagnosis. Within these, the GP may acknowledge the practice processes, their use of consultation skills, or their ethical and knowledge domains which they have brought together to achieve excellence. The annual appraisal is an opportunity for GPs to demonstrate this attainment and continued learning.

An appraiser is allocated by the GP's designated body and there should not be any conflict of interest between the GP and their appraiser; they can't be a friend or practice partner. Appraisals can be completed on paper but almost all of us are using an e-portfolio. There are several services available and the most popular is Clarity, but there is also GPTools (also available for secondary care clinicians) and Fourteen Fish, which has a simple and usable app available (Learning Diary). Clarity uses a traffic light system to show which areas of learning have been completed each appraisal year and revalidation cycle. Every year the GP meets for three hours with their appraiser to run through their learning and development, submitting the e-portfolio two weeks ahead of the meeting. At the end of the meeting, a new personal development plan (PDP) is agreed to for the next 12 months and a 'sign-off' is completed, agreeing to the points discussed during the appraisal. Although appraisals are private and confidential, if the appraiser recognises an issue that causes concern over fitness to practice, this will take precedence over confidentiality and be discussed with the area appraisal lead. After five satisfactory appraisals, the appraiser and appraisal body make a recommendation to the GMC to revalidate the GP as fit to practice. The programme has flexibility for maternity leave, illness and career breaks. Part-time GPs need to provide as much evidence of learning as full-time GPs.

The appraisal is an opportunity to express frustration, discuss disappointment, and to discuss illness in confidence. It is an opportunity to talk about problems within the practice and it is an opportunity for those who are not partners, especially for locums, to receive some GP educator feedback on their professional progression. Annual appraisal is also an opportunity to celebrate personal good practice and practice improvement. It is an opportunity to share achievements and discuss future progression with a GP educator and peer. It can be a great discussion and motivator. The GMC stipulates certain requirements* and the RCGP produces a helpful guide. At present, the evidence of learning constitutes a discussion of the current post and other posts, including evidence of annual appraisals for all posts and a fulfilment of the previous year's PDP. There is also learning (by any method) to a recommended minimum of 50 hours per year and additional practice improvement. This may be a survey and action, a formal audit, a new patient information leaflet, etc. There is discussion of personal significant events and changes required after the GP's critical analysis. Events might be a celebration of excellence, demonstrating use of the latest guidance with good outcomes, or might be an analysis of problems when cases have not gone so well, with action points for improvement. All complaints and compliments should be discussed openly. Within the five-year revalidation cycle the GP should undertake a personal multisource feedback (MSF) to consider the views of peers and teams working with them and a patient satisfaction questionnaire (PSQ).

Annual appraisal encourages personal development through reflective practice and learning, and maintenance of knowledge through continued professional development. It also facilitates reflection of practice through compulsory completion of MSF and PSQ. It ensures a minimum standard of completion of mandatory training in child and adult safeguarding, basic life support, equality and diversity, and information governance.

However, annual appraisals do not observe the GP consulting and cannot fully ensure safe practice. They are time-consuming in a time-stretched job and can feel onerous for some GPs. The choice of mandatory training can seem less of a priority than clinical care and, again, onerous. Many GPs find the reflection aspect difficult to connect with and end up writing platitudes. Reflection is an inner consideration of all aspects of learning with an intent to improve, but it can feel like a personal invasion when exhibited to appraisers. GP trainers and tutors have training on reflection but non-teaching GPs will not always find it easy to do and are more likely to describe outcomes of learning than include processes and emotions of learning and scenarios as an integral part of reflection. That is, reflection should include not only the extrinsic motivators for learning or change but also our intrinsic motivators. Finally, the letter of revalidation can only be described as underwhelming and does not reflect the hard work and excellence of the owner.

Useful resources:

- Royal College of General Practitioners: RCGP Guide to supporting information for appraisal and revalidation (2016) at: http://www.rcgp.org.uk/learning/revalidation/new-revalidation-guidance-for-gps.aspx.
- For GPs experiencing illness the RCGP has a GP wellbeing help and support area to access services at: http://www.rcgp.org.uk/membership/membership-benefits/gp-wellbeing.aspx.

---

* My Appraisal at: http://www.gmc-uk.org/doctors/revalidation.asp

Conclusion

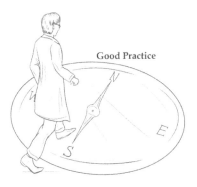

Good Practice

In bringing together the sections of the book, I recommend that you create a mental space in each consultation and I ask you to put on your metaphorical professional white coat. Leave prejudices and behaviours at the consulting room door. The professional coat is surprisingly light and a good fit. Using the skills of consulting, the GP is ready to make best clinical decisions and facilitate the patient.

There are two steps to best decision making. The first is asking the right professional questions and the second is critical analysis for good decision making.

First, ask the right professional questions of yourself and the problem in front of you.

- What do I need to know?
- What is the patient asking?
- How do I find out if I don't know immediately?
- How do I prevent being pushed into immediacy by time pressures and aggressive or coercive behaviour by patients or colleagues?
- Am I asking the right questions of myself; are the answers in my patient's best interests?
- Are there laws and regulations I should explore?
- What are the consultation findings?
- What is the evidence for proposed management plans?
- How does this fit in terms of ethical frameworks and my own professional ethical standing?

Second, use these skills to run the consultation in a professional manner and then to critically analyse all your medical knowledge and the patient's situation. You have brought your knowledge of laws and regulations with you into the consultation to ensure practice is appropriate and current. You have used your consultation skills to gather information about the patient and their presentation. You have your own professional ethics and an ethical framework to analyse the problem presented to you. You have knowledge underpinning your findings and have made a medical best decision but may have alternatives which also have merit. You are now in a position to place your patient in the best position to make their own medical decisions.

As primary care specialists, we GPs now share and contextualise information with our patients in a way that they can comprehend and we contextualize information for them. If we don't do this, be sure the patient will be weighing the choices for themselves. We listen and we personalise the choices they can make in their best interests using critical analysis skills and communication. Decisions may be immediate or delayed; there is not always a rush. Remember that we have our fellow GPs and complete primary care teams working in offices bedside us; we are not isolated even if we feel pressured.

Now the patient can make a good choice.

I hope this book has been an easy read, like slipping a coat on and off, and helps you through the skills and knowledge which we as clinicians take with us into our consulting rooms. I hope you will feel able to put on the coat–your professional skills–more easily after this read. This book is not exhaustive, it is intended as a light read. I don't see this book as author owned; I hope it belongs to everyone. So, if you have comments to improve or resources that are helpful for my next edition please contact jane.wilcock@nhs.net.

We GPs are the profession and we determine its future. If areas of practice need improvement, I urge you to become involved, especially with our college, in a small way so that improvements are by jobbing GPs, affecting real-time patient care and strengthen general practice as a distinct skill set.

Enjoy your general practice and remember: When you take your coat off and go home to relax, you no longer have to give an opinion every 10–15 minutes!

Index